MEDICAL IMPERIALISM IN FRENCH NORTH AFRICA

FRANCE OVERSEAS: STUDIES IN EMPIRE AND DECOLONIZATION

Series editors: A. J. B. Johnston, James D. Le Sueur, and Tyler Stovall

Medical Imperialism in French North Africa

Regenerating the Jewish Community of Colonial Tunis

RICHARD C. PARKS

University of Nebraska Press
LINCOLN AND LONDON

Portions of chapter 2 originally appeared as "*Divide et Impera*: Public Health and Urban Reform in Interwar Tunis" in *Journal of North African Studies* 17, no. 3 (2012): 533–46. Portions of chapter 3 originally appeared as "The Jewish Quarters of Interwar Paris and Tunis: Destruction, Creation, and French Urban Design" in *Jewish Social Studies* 17, no. 1 (Fall 2001): 67–87.

∞

Library of Congress Cataloging-in-Publication Data
Names: Parks, Richard C., author.
Title: Medical imperialism in French North Africa: regenerating the Jewish community of colonial Tunis / Richard C. Parks.
Description: Lincoln: University of Nebraska Press, 2017. | Series: France overseas | Includes bibliographical references and index. |
Identifiers: LCCN 2017011936 (print) |
LCCN 2017013963 (ebook)
ISBN 9781496202871 (epub)
ISBN 9781496202888 (mobi)
ISBN 9781496202895 (pdf)
ISBN 9780803268456 (cloth: alk. paper)
Subjects: LCSH: Jews—Tunisia—Tunis—Social conditions—20th century. | Jews—Health and hygiene—Tunisia—Tunis. | Public health—Tunisia—History—French occupation, 1881–1956. | Tunis (Tunisia)—Social conditions—20th century.
Classification: LCC DS135.T72 (ebook) | LCC DS135.T72 .T867 2017 (print) | DDC 961.10049240904—dc23
LC record available at https://lccn.loc.gov/2017011936

Set in Merope by John Klopping.
Designed by N. Putens.

This book is dedicated to my parents, Clyde and Wanda Parks, who always taught me to value hard work and to be kind to others. And to my sister, Deanna, who is the only person who can make me laugh until I cry.

CONTENTS

MAPS

PREFACE

The benevolent colonizer can never attain the good, for his only choice is not between good and evil, but between evil and uneasiness.

—ALBERT MEMMI, *The Colonizer and the Colonized*

In 1953 Albert Memmi published his first novel, *La statue de sel* (*The Pillar of Salt*), to widespread critical acclaim. The semiautobiographical account, set in the French Protectorate of Tunisia during and after World War II, describes the coming-of-age struggles of Memmi's doppelgänger, Alexandre Mordekhai Benillouche. Although the plotline of the novel is gripping, the value of Memmi's work, as an intellectual and sociohistorical document, lies in the introspective, and often painful, soul-searching of the main character in his quest to define himself in a world of emerging colonial identity politics. As indicated by the character's name (French-Jewish-Tunisian), his persona is splintered among worlds that are increasingly at odds in French-occupied Tunisia. At one point Alexandre contemplates, "I'm a Jew! My home is in the ghetto [*hara*]; my legal status is native African. I'm poor. But I had learnt to reject these four classifications." In fact, the polyvalent, overlapping worlds navigated by Alexandre Mordekhai Benillouche in *The Pillar of Salt* seem to flesh out and make real a world infinitely more complex than the neat dichotomies of "colonizer and colonized" as described and dismantled in Memmi's subsequent nonfiction books, *Portrait du colonisateur* and *Portrait du colonisé* (1957).

The Pillar of Salt grapples not only with the "obviously" problematic categorical juxtapositions of colonizer and colonized, of West and Orient, but it transcends these dichotomies to expose a more nuanced and perilous sociopolitical landscape—a world I view as obsessed with racial, social, and moral regeneration. Through Memmi's skillful narration, we realize that neither the colonizers nor the colonized were monolithic blocs of paralleled interest groups. Within each of these groups were myriad competing religious sects, language groups, political ideologies, and social mores, all of which shaped, to different degrees and at varying times, the identity of each group's members.

My personal interest and involvement in the region go a bit beyond my admiration for the works of Albert Memmi. About twenty years ago, while working as a consultant for the World Bank's Middle East / North Africa department, I became acquainted with the final phases of a plan to "regenerate" parts of the Tunis medina. In the early 1970s the Municipality of Tunis, together with the Association for the Preservation of the Medina (Association de Sauvegarde de la Medina), proposed the urban rehabilitation of nearly fourteen hectares of "abandoned" land in central Tunis. Over the next twenty years, the Tunisian government, with funds provided by the World Bank, cleared the zone of its lingering inhabitants, razed any derelict remains, and built a new quarter of multiuse residential and commercial zones, henceforth known as the Hafsia neighborhood. It was only years later that I made the connection that the "abandoned" land—the site of the newly built Hafsia—was constructed on the destroyed remains of the hara, the Jewish ghetto so vividly described in Memmi's work. For nearly ten centuries, the area in question had been the heart of a thriving Jewish community, and although the hara has been erased from the modern map of Tunis in the most literal sense, traces of a people—the historical flotsam and jetsam of a proud community—linger. My objective is to resituate, reconsider, and reconstruct within the mind's eye the historical events of an intact and imperfect hara and to provide social, cultural, and historical

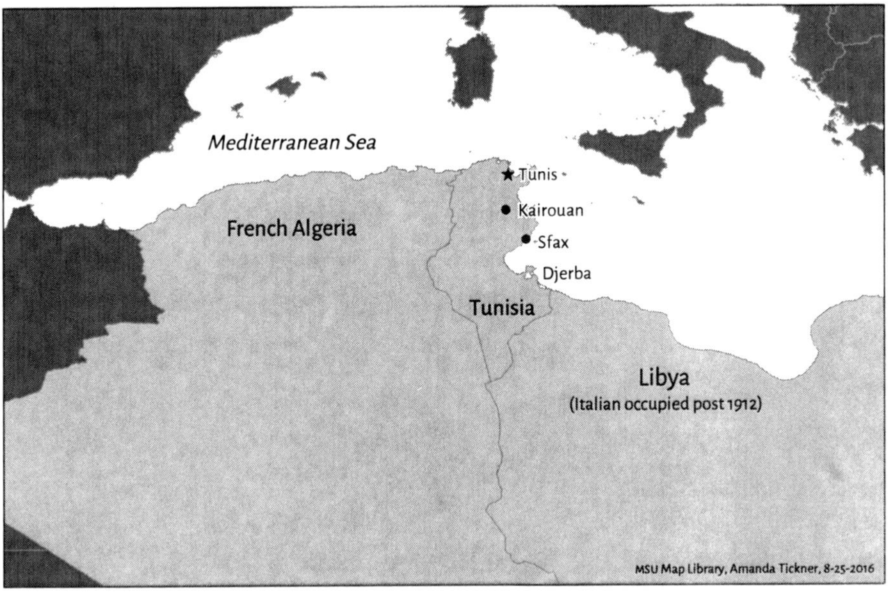

MAP 1. Tunisia and the Maghrib. Created by Amanda Tickner.

context to the world as described by Albert Memmi and as experienced by countless other "colonial subjects."

The final destruction of the Jewish ghetto, and its definitive regeneration as the Muslim-occupied Hafsia, came at the behest of the Tunisian government, which was guided and financed by multinational technocrats. As mentioned, this was not the first time that the hara had been targeted for regeneration. Earlier in the twentieth century, elite members of the Jewish community, both in Tunis and in Paris, led by French-trained public health officials, architects, and city planners, had also called for the destruction and regeneration of the hara. This book examines the events that occurred before and during the finalization of the original plans for the regeneration of the Tunis hara and its people in the early twentieth century. The events recounted and analyzed in this book took place during the waning days of the hara's existence, before the horrors of World War II and the subsequent mass exodus of Jews from the Arab lands of North Africa.

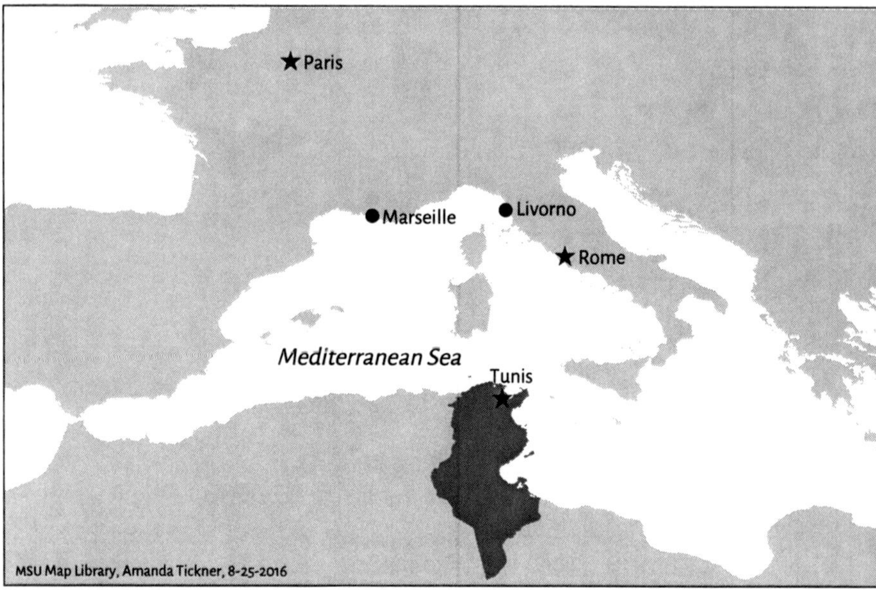

MAP 2. Tunisia in relation to Europe. Created by Amanda Tickner.

Although the original attempts to destroy the Tunis hara that took place in the 1930s exhibit a dramatic manifestation of a community's will to change, the desire to regenerate, remold, and reinvigorate the Jewish community of Tunis went far beyond the demolition of the crumbling remains of an ancient neighborhood—a neighborhood that was, as we shall see, in point of fact incredibly ethnically and religiously diverse. At the heart of this book lies an exploration of the history of the scientific and medical movements and developments of the late nineteenth and early twentieth centuries, almost exclusively French in origin, which, in my view, sparked and sustained the social, cultural, and intellectual will to change Tunis's Jewish community and lead it down the path to regeneration.

ACKNOWLEDGMENTS

I would like to thank Albert Memmi for living a life of inspiration and purpose. I would like to thank my mentors from graduate school at the University of Minnesota, especially Daniel J. Schroeter, who has shown me the greatest kindness and support. I would also like to thank Patricia M. E. Lorcin at Minnesota for her practical guidance, Tamara Giles-Vernick at the Institut Pasteur in Paris for her encouragement when I felt like quitting, and John Eyler for his expertise in the history of medicine. My ideas were able to develop thanks to many avenues of support that have given me the time to research and reflect. I would like to thank the Fulbright Commission, the American Institute for Maghrib Studies (AIMS), the Centre d'Études Maghrébines à Tunis (CEMAT), the Mellon Foundation, the Cogut Center for the Humanities at Brown University, and all of those who have read and commented on drafts of my work.

I would like to thank the librarians and archivists who welcomed me and assisted my research. In France, I would like to thank the Archives de l'Alliance Israélite universelle, the Mémorial de la Shoah, the Archives de l'Institut Pasteur, and the Archives du Ministère des Affaires Étrangères. In Tunis, I would like to thank the Archives nationales de Tunisie, the Institut des Belles Lettres Arabes, the Archives de l'Institut Pasteur de

Tunis, the Pères Blancs, the U.S. Embassy, and the Association de Sauvegarde de la Médina de Tunis. And in the United States, I would like to thank the dedicated archivists at the U.S. Holocaust Memorial Museum and the National Archives.

I would also like to thank the anonymous reviewers of this book for their insightful comments and, of course, the University of Nebraska Press, especially Bridget Barry and her assistant, Emily Wendell, for their guidance. Finishing a book requires the assistance of far too many people and institutions to name. I am grateful to all those who participated in any way toward the completion of this project; you know who you are.

1 Situating Regeneration

Medicine, Science, and "Modern" Bodies

Racism does not limit itself to biology or economics or psychology or metaphysics; it attacks along many fronts and in many forms, deploying whatever is at hand, and even what is not, inventing when the need arises.

— ALBERT MEMMI, *The Colonizer and the Colonized*

In 1857 famed psychologist Bénédict Morel published his highly influential work *Traité des dégénérescences physiques, intellectuelles, et morales de l'espèce humaine* (*Treatise on the Physical, Intellectual and Moral Degeneration of the Human Species*), which identified human degeneration as a scientific reality and valid medical diagnosis. Although written primarily as a psychiatric diagnostic manual, the central theme of Morel's text—human degeneration—held broad appeal as a scientific explanation for a host of late nineteenth- and early twentieth-century woes. On one hand, degeneration described and explained the social upheavals provoked by the Industrial Revolution and settler colonialism, both situations in which society's elites had daily contact with the inherently degenerate masses. But on the other hand, the theory of degeneration also warned that the perils of degeneration were not consigned exclusively to the slums of the lumpen proletariat and the disordered world of the colonial subject.

Degeneration, as an ontological category, also implicated the "modern condition" as a threat to the fragility of the cultivated Western body and mind and created a new category of dysfunction to encompass intellectual, physical, and moral deficiencies, both real and imagined.

Morel, with his novel diagnosis of degeneration, was part of a burgeoning school of French psychiatrists and pathologists who sought to identify mental and physical disorders through scientific empiricism. But in a broader sense, Morel and his fellow alienists were emblematic of a larger movement of clinically trained specialists who sought answers to complex medical problems in both the controlled environment of the laboratory and the tumult of the mental asylum, through the observation of live subjects and postmortem autopsies, using both qualitative data and statistical evidence. According to this new school of experts, the pursuit of knowledge was no longer "academic," it served a practical point: to identify and eliminate the characteristic evils of modern society.

More and more, Western society placed its trust in science and medicine to provide a wellspring of answers to life's complex and hitherto intractable problems. According to this line of thinking, once informed by the unimpeachable authority of scientific and medical knowledge, states would govern more effectively, cities would be cleansed, and experts would manage rationally life's most mundane decisions. The emergence of "new sciences," such as statistics, microbiology, urban planning, and sanitation (to name but a few), shifted the onus of finding answers to an exclusive cadre of experts. In France a new technocratic elite trained exclusively to manage the complexities of quotidian existence emerged from the *grandes écoles*—École Normale Supérieur, École Polytechnique, and the Conservatoire National des Arts et Métiers—(re)conceived in the wake of the Revolution of 1789. Following a rather circular train of logic, successive French regimes tasked the new technocratic elite with finding modern scientific and medical solutions to the lurking dangers of degeneration, a disease that ironically found much of its origin in man's struggle with modernity. For the most part, it was easy for scientists and physicians to wrap their minds around the degenerative maladies associated with modernity: the stresses of the terrible rumble of train travel, the exasperating hurly-burly of increased urban population, and the stench and filth associated with large concentrations of industrial machinery and laborers. These omnipresent facets of modern life caused the common signs of degeneration seen in the middle and upper classes: neurasthenia, hysteria, alcoholism, homosexuality, epilepsy, effeteness, and narcissism.[1] But it was the inherent racial and attendant class-based manifestations of degeneration that were more difficult to pinpoint and that required more extensive and elaborate explications.

As settler colonialism brought white Europeans into close, daily contact with indigenous peoples and industrialization brought the upper classes into more direct contact with the proletariat, science became hard-pressed to elaborate theories to explain human difference: how the white, bourgeois mind and body differed from that of the "natives" or the "working classes." Moreover, Enlightenment scholars, obsessed with the classification and categorization of the natural world, including human "types," struggled to explain scientifically the large amount of phenotypic variation present in the human species. Western science assumed with little or no debate the fact that Europeans would take a preeminent position at the summit of the racial hierarchy. To the vast majority of these scholars, the notion that "whites" were superior to "blacks," or to any other colonized population for that matter, was a given—the issue at hand was how to furnish scientific justifications in support of this apparent fact. Philosophers, scientists, and dilettantes alike offered a wide variety of explanations for racial phenotypic variation, ranging from biblical accounts of Noah's wayward (and racially diverse) sons to Voltaire's Hippocratic-based theories of climactic adaptation. How and why the races were somatically different were hotly debated, but the learned consensus of experts maintained that the white European was special. Still, even within the specialness of European whiteness, there were gradations among those who best represented the inherent virtues of the *Homo europeaus*. Few disputed that fact that the highborn and the wealthy possessed qualities superior to those of the lower classes in much the same way that the races themselves differed.[2]

Racial purity, however one chose to justify it, was a highly unstable category. Inherent in any argument seeking to validate and promote the supremacy of the white, wealthy European race was the fear of racial contamination and the subsequent dissolution of the European species. Racial theorists cum anthropologists, like Johann Blumenbach and the Comte de Buffon, posited that the dilution of "pure" races through miscegenation exacerbated the spreading scourge of racial decay.[3] Europeans were expected to abide by the visual signposts that nature had erected between the races and to respect the phenotypic barriers between the "white" European, "black" African, and "yellow" Asiatic. However, some race experts noted that lurking within the liminal spaces of phenotypic and inherent biological difference, among white, black, and yellow, there existed another special classification of human typology, the "Jewish race," which was already present and living among the European species. Although ostensibly "white" and "European," Jews, even those of the upper classes, presented a unique challenge to those obsessed with racial classification and concerned about the perils of degeneration. These obsessions with the race and class of European Jews, and their capacity for regeneration, held important implications, as we will see, for Tunisian Jews.

The Medical Tradition

But before we continue the discussion about degeneration, regeneration, and racial science, it is helpful to revisit the unique and enduring history of scientific and medical exchange that existed between Europe and the Arab world, which helps to explain the ease with which many in the Tunisian community embraced late nineteenth- and early twentieth-century medical theories in regard to eugenic degeneration. For more than a millennium, educated physicians in Europe, the Maghrib, and the Middle East, whether Jewish, Christian, or Muslim, had accepted the major tenets of the medical texts passed down from classical Greece and Rome as enhanced during the golden age of Islam at Baghdad's House of Wisdom (Ar. Bayt al-Hikma). From these classical sources, philosopher physicians learned environmental and holistic theories of disease etiology and therapeutics as explained in the case studies of the Hippocratic treatises dating from 400 BCE. Carefully recorded clinical notes and empirical research guided successive generations of healers whose results were compiled into a corpus of medical knowledge. To the philosophical and empirical foundations of the ancient Greeks, the Ptolemaic Greeks, Herophilos, Erasistratus, and others of the Alexandrian school of medicine added their knowledge of gross anatomy, including a mapping of the veins, arteries, and nervous system in the third century BCE.

But much of the foundation of the humoral medicine that would come to dominate learned understandings of the human body is credited to the second-century Greco-Roman philosopher Galen, who combined the teachings of Aristotelian philosophy, Hippocratic empiricism, and Alexandrian anatomical research to articulate the theoretical prototype of human health and well-being. The primary tenet of Galenic humoral medicine, like its Hippocratic predecessor, is based on idiopathic equilibrium: each body has a natural state of balance of its hot, wet, cold, and dry humors, which is tantamount to good health. Disturbance of this unique and natural humoral balance results in disease. According to Galen, only a learned philosopher-physician possessed the required knowledge to recalibrate the diseased body's imbalance through diet, exercise, and of course, bloodletting and cautery, which were all highly dependent on other interrelated factors, such as season, temperament, and astrology.

The intricate medical system built on Galen's theories of humoral medicine would likely have died out with the fall of the Roman Empire had it not been for their widespread adoption outside the boundaries of the shrinking empire, first in Byzantium and later in the rapidly expanding world of Islam. In fact, much of the Greco-Roman traditions, on which Christendom claimed to be founded, had been lost or forgotten by European scholars in the chaos of the collapse of the Roman Empire and the subsequent "barbarian" invasions. But in the Early Middle Ages, Jewish and Muslim scholars from Umayyad al-Andalus reintroduced the textual history of ancient Greece and Rome to medieval Europe, including the tenets of learned Galenic medicine and Greco-Roman philosophy.

Although medievalists debate the degree to which Jews were accepted as part of the Islamic community in Umayyad Iberia, there is little doubt that Jews played an integral role in the translation and dissemination of medical and philosophical texts, not only within the world of Islam, but also in Christendom.[4] Jews, as a "homeless" diasporic people who were found within the realms of both Christendom and Islam, became important arbiters and agents of cross-cultural exchange who reintroduced to Western Europeans the philosophical underpinnings of humoral theory, diagnosis, therapeutics, and pharmacopeia, which had been safely harbored and enhanced greatly in the Arab world.

In short Jews, Muslims, and Christians, in spite of their political and religious differences, shared common philosophical precepts in regard to the physiological, and even spiritual, functions of the human body. This familiarity of terms and a sharing of common concepts eased the way for the transmission of ideas between Europe and the Maghrib, including the new concepts of racial difference and regeneration that surfaced in the nineteenth and twentieth centuries. It is true that local communities in the Maghrib practiced various types of Islamic medicine, Prophetic medicine (Ar. *al-Tibb al-nabawii*), or Jewish medicine, but each of these medical paradigms shares common roots in Greek philosophy, Galenic humoral tradition, and healing customs also practiced on the European side of the Mediterranean. Although the reception of ideas in the Maghrib was not seamless, it is undeniable that principles of physiology, philosophies of medicine, and scientific mind-sets were exchanged across the Mediterranean Sea with a facility that was not seen when Western medicine arrived in areas with dramatically different cosmological explications of the human body and its well-being, like sub-Saharan Africa or Far East Asia.

In spite of the intellectual debt of gratitude owed to the Orient, much religious and political antagonism lingered among Jews, Muslims, and Christians well into the modern era, and European Christians harshly persecuted Jews in their midst. Before the Enlightenment, when most Europeans—or at least, those who valued their lives and reputations—viewed intellectual thought and scientific advancement through the sanctioned, narrow prism of Catholicism, there was little room for dissent in regard to spiritual beliefs and religious dogma. The Catholic Church dominated political, social, and even economic life in Europe, and Jews were spurned and persecuted as a religious sect that refused to accept the "one true faith." Although the Reformation created a chink in the armor of papal authority, the one thing on which the feuding sects of Protestantism and Catholicism could agree was the disapprobation of Jews. Unlike the infidel and the pagan—or the Protestant in the eyes of those who remained loyal to Rome—European Jews embodied a stubborn and long-standing religious apostasy within the confines of Christendom. Christians, regardless of sectarian difference or internecine warfare, agreed that Jews were abhorrent and aberrant in their rejection of the message of Jesus Christ as the Son of God.

Jews in France

As religious influence waned during the Enlightenment, especially in France, which saw the power and prestige of the Catholic Church diminished even further by the subsequent violence of the Revolution, intellectuals posited that French secularism, in jettisoning the yoke of Rome, similarly shot down attendant ideas of Jewish "difference" based on religious apostasy. However, this secular laissez-faire attitude of acceptance proved to be a mixed blessing for Jews. As the religious impediments to acceptance were being systematically dismantled, the continuation of Jewish exclusion in continental Europe increasingly relied on the *racial* difference of the Jew, now defined as an inherent somatic condition that religious otherness only aggravated. The expanded reliance on science and medicine to explain racial disparities, together with the secularization of Jewish difference led to new theories of redemption for the Jewish body. In this new view, revitalization and "regeneration" of Jews would not necessarily stem from conversion to Christianity; the path to salvation lay increasingly within the purview of science and medicine. Indeed, as regarded Jews, the focus had shifted in the French mind from saving souls to regenerating bodies.

One of the earliest manifestations of this new focus can be seen in the philosophical and political writings of Abbé Henri Grégoire. In 1788, in response to a scholastic competition, Abbé Henri Grégoire presented to the Royal Society of France his famous essay advocating the redemption and "regeneration" of French Jews.[5] Igniting much controversy, the abbé publicly stated that the Creator had endowed Jews with certain sociopolitical rights and that Jews, once rescued from their degenerate state, could and should be incorporated into the fabric of French society.[6] In 1789 Abbé Grégoire became the official representative for Jews at the newly reconvened Estates General at Versailles, and his advocacy for Jewish inclusion laid the cornerstone for equality and French citizenship.[7]

In an effort to normalize relations between Jews and Christians in France, one of the primary goals of a newly emerging Franco-Jewish elite was to battle degeneration within their fold. In the eyes of the French state, unto which a Jewish consistory became an official arm in 1808, the nineteenth-century social transformation of France's Jewish community was a remarkable success.[8] The Franco-Jewish community, especially those concentrated in large, urban areas, like Paris, Strasbourg, and Bordeaux, increasingly found a home in the liberal professions, the military, the government, and French social and cultural life in a broader sense. Although the tolerance of French Jews was not entirely universal, by the mid-nineteenth century, the community enjoyed a level of acceptance and absorption into the social, cultural, and political makeup of their nation unrivaled in continental Europe. The successful integration and acculturation of French Jews became a template for other European nations but also for the French imperial administration, which was rapidly acquiring foreign territories with substantial indigenous Jewish populations.

In 1860, encouraged by the successful incorporation of Jews into French society and concerned for the "Oriental" Jews in the growing French Empire, famed statesman Adolphe Crémieux founded the Alliance Israélite Universelle (AIU) in Paris with the express aim of "regenerating" the Jews of the Mediterranean basin.[9] The regenerating efforts of the AIU focused almost entirely on the supremacy of French culture, civilization, and political freedom of expression to act as reformative influences in colonial Jewish communities. The AIU became a powerful force in the dissemination of French values and advocated a straightforward formula of cultural and social assimilation as the most successful means of regeneration. After France acquired its "Oriental" empire, much of its Jewish population, backed by the power of the French state's colonial apparatus, shifted its attention from the introspective scrutiny of French Jews to a thoroughgoing consideration of the taxonomy of colonial "Arab" Jews. Harnessing the power of the biological, sociocultural, and political classifications inherent in the science of race, metropolitan forces were now poised to effect the regeneration of an entirely new segment of global French society: the colonized Jew.

"Tunisian" Jews

The unique characteristics and widely divergent origins of Maghribi Jewish communities defied the traditional strictures of European racial classification. Tunisian Jews, as "African" Jews, were difficult to pigeonhole neatly into discrete taxonomical and sociocultural groups within preexisting historical, anthropological, and racial narratives. Even today, the fact that the Maghrib is a "border zone" that occupies various geographical and historical planes (Europe, Africa, the Middle East, and the Mediterranean) complicates the ability of scholars to analyze the important history of the Maghrib and Tunisian Jews.[10]

Shifting political and religious boundaries and significant long-distance population migration call into question the use of the deceptively vague descriptor "Tunisian Jews" to designate a community that existed long before the political or cartographical existence of Tunisia.[11] The power to name groups of people and to determine the social, political, and geographical parameters of their identities is a tricky business that bestows considerable power into the hands of historians. The stalwart though misguided contemporary conviction that identity corresponds at least implicitly to the nation-state paradigm, coupled with the facility of anachronistic thinking, often blinds us to alternative constructions and expressions of group identity and the ways in which these identities develop and change over the *longue durée*. The subjectivity of identity in addition to its historical ephemerality requires careful definitions and precision as to the meanings and parameters of group identity markers. Within this book's late nineteenth- and early twentieth-century purview, the Tunisian Jewish identity was a *colonial identity* with all of the resultant ambiguities, tensions, and unrequited aspirations inherent in the colonial experience.[12]

When the French seized control of Tunisia, there were two competing Jewish identities in mainland Tunisia, Twansa and Grana, whose histories are central to the ultimate realization of the Tunisian Jewish colonial "regenerationist" identity. There has been much debate among historians and anthropologists as to the veracity of local lore, which asserts that the long history of Jews in modern-day Tunisia stretches back to the pre-Roman era. The traditional claims that Jews arrived in Tunisia with the founding of Carthage (874 BCE) or after the destruction of the First Temple in the sixth century BCE remain historically unsubstantiated, but incontrovertible evidence of a synagogue and a Jewish cemetery in Tunisia can be documented by the third century CE.[13] Between this initial fledgling settlement of Jews in Tunisia and the seventh century CE, various Roman, Vandal, and Byzantine era "Europeans," as well as some indigenous seminomadic tribesmen converted to Judaism.[14] Conversions to Judaism came to a halt at the end of the seventh century, when Arab Muslims conquered Tunisia (Ar. al-Ifriqiya) and transformed Tunis, which is uniquely protected from naval attack by Lake Tunis (lac de Tunis), into a port that gave easy access both to the western Mediterranean and the Italian Peninsula. At this time, the late seventh century, the Umayyad conquerors also founded the city of Kairouan (Ar. al-Quyrawan) about a hundred miles to the south of Tunis. Kairouan grew to become a great center of Islamic and Jewish learning with the largest concentration of Jews in the Maghrib. In the tenth and eleventh centuries, the Kairouan Jewish community, led by a strong hierarchical community structure, was second only to the Jews of Baghdad in terms of spiritual and intellectual vigor.[15] Very little is known in regard to the Jewish community between this highpoint of Kairouan and the horrors of the Almohad era (1160–1229 CE), which witnessed rampant persecution and forced conversion of Jews. In 1229 Abu Zakariya Yahya ousted the Almohads and began the three-and-a-half-century reign of the Hafsid dynasty (1229–1574 CE).

Under Hafsid rule Tunis emerged as the capital of the Hafsid kingdom and asserted its role as a burgeoning center of trade with Christian European and other Mediterranean ports. Hafsid rule ushered in a time of relative peace and prosperity for Jews in Tunisia—greater than that enjoyed by any other Jewish community in the Maghrib—and Jews began to settle in greater numbers in Tunis, many relocating from Kairouan.[16] Islam considered Jews as "people of the book" and deemed *"ahl al-dhimma,"* or "protected people," which allowed them to practice their religion contingent on the acceptance of certain legal disabilities. Over the many years of Jewish-Islamic cohabitation, Jews shared their daily lives with their Islamic neighbors and developed strategies of mutual coexistence, including common economic, linguistic, and cultural ties. It is probably during the Hafsid era that Jews in Tunis adopted the moniker "Twansa," meaning "from Tunis." The Twansa identity, limited to Tunis at first, expanded outward from Tunis and by the Ottoman era referred more generally to "indigenous Jews."

In the late fifteenth century, the arrival of Sephardic Jews expelled from Iberia transformed the ethnic and sociocultural composition of many Jewish communities in North Africa; however, Tunisia received far fewer Spanish and Portuguese Jews than did Morocco or Algeria. More significant for Tunisia was the arrival of mercantile port Jews, two centuries later, from the Tuscan trading harbor of Livorno.[17] Livorno, a duty-free haven under the control of Tuscany's Medici clan, had thrived for more than a century by accepting merchant outcasts, usually Jews and Protestants, from elsewhere in Europe. In the late seventeenth century, Livornese Jews, eager to expand their trade network, settled in significant numbers in "satellite" Mediterranean port cities, like Tunis.[18] Elite, expatriate Livornese Jews formed lucrative commercial linkages between cities like Tunis, Amsterdam, and Salonika and the Jewish community back in Tuscany. These satellite communities of Livornese Jews formed "a distinct social group within a Jewish community, . . . living side by side with other Jews who were not 'port Jews' in the social and cultural sense of the term."[19]

Once Jews from "outside" began to arrive in Tunis in significant numbers in the late seventeenth century, there was additional reason to have terminology differentiating "indigenous Jews," or "Twansa," from the new arrivals. Henceforth, the Livornese Jews in Tunis were known to indigenous Twansa Jews as "Grana," a term derived from al-Ghurna, the Arabic name for Livorno, and also slang for "Portuguese," in reference to the assumed native roots of Grana Jews in the Iberian Peninsula. In the Twansa community, the terms *"Grana," "Portuguese,"* and *"Livornese"* were fluid and interchangeable, and the moniker *juif portugais* became a universal term for Sephardic Jews from Western Europe, in much the same way that continental Italians referred to all Iberian Jews, regardless of exact provenance, as *ebrei spagnoli* (Spanish Jews).

Grana Jews were acculturated to European values and differentiated themselves from the Twansa by maintaining the Judeo-Italian vernacular known as *bagitto* or *bagito*, which they had brought with them from Livorno.[20] For their part, the Twansa spoke a distinctive Judeo-Arabic dialect, which in addition to its Hebrew vocabulary elements differed phonologically from the Muslim vernacular.[21] From the late sixteenth century until the late eighteenth century, Tunis thrived as a commercial hub and became rich from the booty of corsairs and the ransoms obtained from families of captured European sailors. The most elite Grana Jews with commercial ties to other important port cities formed a cadre of traders, bankers, and government officials in Tunisia who participated in Tunis's expanding economic influence. Twansa Jews, and less well-connected Grana Jews, worked as artisans and craftsmen: tailors, goldsmiths, jewelers, cobblers, and carpenters. Although a few families accumulated prodigious wealth, the majority of Jews in Tunis, both Grana and Twansa, lived in relative poverty.[22]

Social, cultural, and religious interaction between the newly arrived Grana Jews and the indigenous Twansa Jews was strained and limited. The Grana established an autonomous community in 1710, with separate synagogues, cemeteries, and marketplace (Ar. *Sūq al-Grana*). The schism was made official in 1741 with an agreement signed by the leading rabbis of the rival sects. While there were divisions and disputes elsewhere in North Africa where European Sephardim settled, the Grana community's most controversial act in Tunisia was the establishment of its own kosher slaughterhouse that controlled the taxes levied on butchered meat. Twansa Jews accused the Grana of eschewing their financial responsibilities to the larger Jewish community. The rift between the Grana and Twansa, which lasted for nearly two hundred years, was one of economic resentment and cultural disconnect.[23] Grana Jews, in spite of their proximity to the Twansa Jewish community, remained aloof. Twansa Jews shared their space and port with Grana Jews, but the gulf between the two communities guaranteed that Enlightenment philosophy, secular reforms, and acculturation to European life, widely accepted by most Grana, remained alien concepts to most in the Twansa community until introduced by the French Protectorate.

When the French wrested control of Tunisia from Bey Muhammad al-Sadiq in 1881, it is safe to say that there was not a hegemonic Tunisian Jewish identity within the geographical and political confines of the newly established protectorate.[24] Although Twansa Jews had formed an expanding, though loosely demarcated community since the Regency of Tunis, the influx of Grana Jews followed by the shock of French military and political interventionism shattered preexisting boundaries and created a political and sociocultural void within the Tunisian Jewish community as a whole. Within this space, a new colonial identity forged in the crucible of imperial expansionism was created. The Tunisian Jewish colonial identity, as we shall see, was a modern identity at the core of which lay the determination to regenerate oneself through rationalization, secularization, reformation, acculturation, or civilization—all of which, as this book demonstrates, rested implicitly or explicitly on a scaffold of scientific and medical authority.

However, by naming a Tunisian Jewish colonial identity, I do not mean to imply that all Jews in Tunisia were united "under one flag" or that they shared a political ideology within our understanding of allegiance to the nation-state. On the contrary, Tunisian Jewish colonial identity was unevenly adopted and manifested itself through myriad social customs, group memberships, and allegiances. But under the auspices of the colonial regime, the message of secular education and emancipation through Western acculturation, which had already taken root in the Grana community, received a warm reception in the Twansa community as well. The French protectorate leveled the playing field between the two factions and encouraged, often unwittingly, new modes of collaborative Jewish expression, like Zionism.

Several phenomena explain the relative ease with which Tunisian Jews, Twansa and Grana, latched onto the colonial identity. Twansa Jews responded positively to an identity that promised emancipation, a safeguard from abuses, and the potential for all to prosper; rights that were already ostensibly granted to their Grana brethren. As a community defined by their socioeconomic prowess, Grana Jews expressed waning concern in shifting their allegiance from Italy to the French regime once power dynamics in the Mediterranean had changed in France's favor. Another important factor in the broad acceptance of the Tunisian Jewish colonial identity is that neither Grana Jews nor Twansa Jews defined their community through the paradigm of a romanticized Andalusian past.[25] The Grana identity, as a diasporic merchant community, was elastic enough to allow for a shift in political allegiance, from Italy to France, so long as the underlying political and socioeconomic protections remained intact. Adherence to a new colonial identity based on "civil inclusion" or "*Haskalah avant la lettre*," to which they were already accustomed, required a modification of national loyalty, not acquiescence to a new way of life.[26] Once that shift began, Grana Jews became powerful allies to the French forces tasked with disseminating the civilizing mission of regeneration to indigenous Twansa Jews.[27]

The Science of Race

In 1862, just after the founding of the AIU and on the eve of the dramatic expansion of France's African empire, the French translation of Darwin's groundbreaking book *On the Origin of Species*, which purported, among other things, to explain the origins of man and his place in the natural world, was published.[28] The elaboration of the theories of evolution and natural selection, with their implication of constant species' adaptation and existential struggle, indelibly influenced the tenor of the regenerationist crusade. From this point forward, regeneration was set loose from its social and political moorings and launched into the sea of scientific and medical discourse—regeneration, race science, and eugenics would be forevermore inextricably linked.[29] Although the AIU cautiously tailored its regenerative message to incorporate the scientific and medical authority of Darwinism and eugenics, the organization remained committed to its reliance on the redemptive strength of sociocultural assimilation. On the other hand, Zionism, which emerged at the end of the nineteenth century, was far more skilled and proficient in using the medical and scientific aspects of eugenics as the handmaiden of Jewish regeneration.

Although the historiographical record portrays Jews almost exclusively as the victims of the horrors of race science and eugenics, the actual history of the intersection of race science, eugenics, and Jews presents a more nuanced account.[30] During the apogee of French imperial control in the Maghrib, from the Belle Époque to the dawn of World War II, most Jewish scientists, physicians, and social reformers, whether proponents of the AIU's "civilizing" approach or the Zionists more "technical" methods, viewed eugenics, which relied on a view of Lamarckian trait heritability and human plasticity that was unique to French circles, as a means to perfect the Jewish race. According to Lamarck's theory of heritability, traits acquired during one's lifetime, whether negative or positive, could be passed to one's offspring. In simple terms, a couple that sought intellectual pursuits and remained physically fit would bear intelligent and healthy children. In its most extreme iteration, a blacksmith could pass to his sons the bulging muscles developed by the swing of his hammer or an accountant could pass along his strong mathematical ability to figure accounts rapidly and accurately. The optimism of this theory is that the heritability of newly acquired traits is immediate and demonstrable. Therefore, the "reformed woman" rescued from the viciousness of drink and prostitution could bear worthy children. A weak and downtrodden man who took to physical fitness could produce strong children. The possibilities for self-improvement, and hence improvement of the race or species, were manifold.

From its inception, eugenics in France was understood and practiced very differently than it was the rest of the Western world.[31] Although many scientists in the international community during the nineteenth century explained and understood Darwinian theory through some form of Lamarckian heritability, none were as optimistic as the French. For obvious reasons, the optimism of French eugenics, which opened the door of opportunity to the most downtrodden of society, appealed to French Jews and, moreover, presented itself as a concept ready-made for colonial consumption. Conversely, scientists in the United States, Great Britain, Germany, and Sweden continued to view eugenics through the pessimistic prism of racial purity and focused on ways to forbid or prevent the dilution of qualities inherent to the Anglo-Teutonic race.[32] Eugenics in these nations meant that science and the state should work hand in glove to identify "carriers" of vicious, negative traits and then erect barriers to prevent these individuals from breeding. In dramatic contrast, French officials, no doubt motivated by the flagging national birthrate, especially after the defeat of French forces at the hands of the Prussians in 1871, emphasized pronatalist policies and a newfound fixation on puericulture. France urged its citizens to have more, not fewer, children. In the highly Lamarckian French view, "undesirable" traits could be winnowed out over the course of a lifetime; hence, only the more desirable traits that were promoted by governmental and scientific tutelage would be transferred to subsequent generations. As the Anglo-Saxon and Germanic nations enacted programs to restrict immigration and eliminate the "unfit" from the national population, the focus in France was on increasing both the quality *and* the quantity of births.[33]

The gulf between the Anglo-Germanic and French approaches widened even more at the dawn of the twentieth century, when the scientific community rediscovered Gregor Johann Mendel's mid-nineteenth-century pea plant experiments that demonstrated fixed and specific patterns of trait heritability. Mendel's research showed that trait heritability was not "blended" as originally thought but followed patterns dictated by the recessive or dominant nature of a given trait. In short Mendel's experiments disproved Lamarckian heritability. Regardless of these findings, which were widely accepted by the majority of the international scientific community, French science stubbornly clung to Lamarckian ideas of trait heritability. Whether the French were motivated by national pride in Lamarck or just the "commonsense" appeal of his theories is subject to debate.[34] More important to the purposes of my argument is that the French held a unique view of the link between the regenerative benefits of self-improvement—which dovetailed conveniently with widespread, lingering beliefs in Saint-Simonianism—and the fitness of future generations.[35] This expansive view of regeneration, which circulated throughout the Jewish community in France, and ultimately Tunisia, was an interpretation that was not necessarily measured in terms of biological or somatic change. The effects and manifestations of regeneration among the Jews of Tunis could *also* be gauged by such factors as cultural growth, material urban reform, or quite simply an acknowledgment of and adaptation to the superiority of French "modernity" and savoir faire.

As French imperial control expanded its territorial limits from Algeria to Tunisia, and finally to Morocco, elites in France and the Maghrib, Jews and Christian alike, pondered the ways in which the sociocultural "normalization" of Jewish-Christian relations in the metropole and the attendant promises of regeneration could be harnessed and exported in order to acculturate the newly acquired colonial populations of "Oriental" Jews. The seeds of regeneration, introduced under the guise of acculturation and normalization, which had taken firm root in mainland France, found fertile soil in the Jewish communities of the Maghrib.

The social positivism of the nineteenth century fed a belief in biological determinism that supported the preconceived notions of protectorate officials and metropolitan audiences in regard to the "natives" of the Maghrib. French officials expressed little interest in modernizing or regenerating the Muslim community, which they regarded as inherently "unassimilable natives" predisposed to irrationality, fatalism, and self-segregation.[36] Metropolitan and protectorate authorities considered the alleged laziness and fatalism of Muslims as indelible biological traits that would be difficult, perhaps impossible, to weed out. On the other hand, neo-Lamarckian beliefs in the mutability of heritable traits did sustain a degree of optimism in the ability of the French to regenerate the Maghrib. This was especially true for Jews, who, according to the theories of the age, had shown themselves to be a highly adaptable race, able to conform themselves with great elasticity to myriad social and environmental climes. French indifference toward Muslims but inclusion of Jews in the colonial regenerationist schemes was likely based on several interrelated factors. First, there was already an established metropolitan tradition of attempts to modernize and assimilate Jews into the national fabric of France dating back to the late eighteenth-century work of Abbé Grégoire.[37] Second, a strong metropolitan lobby of Jews, best represented by the "founding fathers" of the AIU, transported this idea of Jewish acculturation and "rehabilitation" to the colonial environment.[38] And lastly, Muslims, unlike their Jewish neighbors, lacked an influential metropolitan presence that could lobby for the interests of their coreligionists.

The dubious quest for "modernity" was among the most insidious aspects of colonial domination.[39] *Medical Imperialism in French North Africa* considers the ways in which the Jewish community grappled with regeneration as a reactionary movement obsessed with demarcating the limits and definitions of French colonial modernity and modern identity. The word "modern," which derives from the Latin *modernus* via the Old French *moderne* (ca. 1450–1500), originally meant "just now" or "every day" and was used to form a temporal juxtaposition to what had come before or had already passed. But by the late nineteenth and early twentieth centuries, the definitions of "modern" and "modernity" as linguistic terms had undergone a dramatic transformation. As the West expanded and interacted with world communities, the meaning of "modern" morphed into the perfect foil to describe what Europe was, in relation to everything it supposedly was not: primitive, irrational, backward, and superstitious.[40] This assumed cultural superiority, laced with heavy overtones of eugenic purity, was not exclusive to the French but existed in countless circumstances in which the West came in contact with indigenous people—any instance in which Western superiority was defined by its antithesis: "native."[41] Western Enlightenment notions of alterity were formed by the very colonial encounters they sought to describe.[42] Western expansion and colonialism reshaped modernity into a universalizing concept used to highlight social exclusions and reify the dominance of cultural constructions of difference. Although the "other" is considered as part of the modern narrative, the "other" is still not central enough to be considered constitutive.[43] Backward cultures produce no ideas, goods, or services that the modern world desires—with one notable exception: the exotic. "Modern" and the "modern other" became subjective terms, and myriad motives and factors—social, cultural, economic, political—helped shape this subjectivity. My aim is to interrogate these Western claims of modernity and supremacy, at least as it concerns the limited case of Tunisian Jews in the French Maghrib.

Part and parcel of colonial modernity was a formation of hybrid categories of social and cultural identity and belonging. To some scholars, cultural hybridity is a construction that assumes and reifies Western claims of superiority—the native mimics his overlord. However, if we reject built-in assumptions of Eurocentrism and Western supremacy, we can shift the "contact zone" of hybrid culture from the colony back to the metropole itself, or perhaps to a neutral third space.[44] My work demonstrates that in many respects the formation of social and cultural hybrid identity was dialectical and simultaneously located in metropolitan space.[45] Often, iterations and applications of modernity were witnessed in colonial space long before their implementation in the metropole.[46] The elaboration of colonial modernity was an ever-changing, highly contingent sociohistorical process predicated on innumerable intersections between the metropole and the periphery. These discrete, yet critical encounters between the French colonizers and the Tunisian Jewish community lie at the heart of understanding regeneration.[47]

Historians are trained to view with a gimlet eye the assertion that all "modern" knowledge (scientific, medical, cultural, etc.) emanated outward from the metropole and either took root or withered in the virgin soil of colonial space—that the colonies acted as a passive repository or recipient of European knowledge but contributed little or no value in their own right.[48] In French colonial Africa, historians have struggled to determine whether the colonies acted as a laboratory for sociocultural and scientific experimentation, as a recipient of civilizing and regenerative ideas already tested and validated in the metropole, or more likely, as a bit of both.[49] Framing new inquiries with the latter most of these choices in mind shifts the historical question in a way that allows for considerations of colonial agency, coordination, and cooperation in the regenerative schemes that were hatched for the "good of the colonized." This approach also avoids reducing the colonies to the status of a passive vessel and congratulating Europe as the font of all useful knowledge.

As historian Alice Conklin has stated, "The colonies were never just laboratories; they were sites, however unequal, of conflict and negotiation between colonizer and colonized, where French assumptions about the ability of Africans to evolve, and of France to civilize them, were contested and periodically reshaped."[50] In fact, many of the ideas that directly impinged on regeneration and modern identity in French colonial Tunisia did not originate in the metropole. In countless examples, as this book shows, novel ideas were not imposed on the colonies; rather, the conception, development, and promotion of the ideas bounced back and forth between colony and metropole in an elaborate intellectual discussion shaped by hopes, desires, political influence, and material realities. Any and all form(s) of modernity(ies) in colonial Tunisia, including ideas about "regeneration," inferred both the deconstruction of the sociocultural paradigm that had preceded it and the reconstitution of a new sociocultural order.[51] The dismantlement and reconfiguration of this order in French colonial Tunisia spawned the creation of a Tunisian Jewish colonial identity regenerated through the authority of science and medicine. This book presents brief but meaningful vignettes of how French officials and colonial subjects in the French Protectorate of Tunisia, chiefly within Tunis's Jewish community, transformed the powerful rhetoric of regeneration and concomitant beliefs related to modernity and identity into operational projects buttressed by the unimpeachable authority of science and medicine. Spearheaded by the AIU and proponents of Zionism, regeneration, as a blueprint to rescue and rehabilitate, was somewhat unique to colonized Jewish communities, although countless analogous schemes bearing such names as "the civilizing mission" (*mission civilisatrice*), "assimilation," "association," and "the white man's burden" flourished throughout the colonized world.[52]

Understanding the forces that shaped sociocultural and political identity in the colonial world and the impact of these forces on colonial policy is a central concern to historians and anthropologists. Scholars of the French Empire have zeroed in on the unfulfilled promise of universal citizenship and the duplicitous nature of the French "civilizing mission." Scholarship aimed at fleshing out the parameters of colonial identity under the French imperial project has raised broader questions and insinuations important to this study, namely, that the colonial other represented a "degenerate species." In our quest to understand the reception and spread of the rhetoric of regeneration and modern identity in colonial space, it is important to remember that these efforts were "simultaneously universalizing and particularizing . . . at once republican and illiberal."[53]

Obsessive academic focus on the archival narrative, which privileges the voice of the colonizer, and individual motives of colonial administrators can *perhaps* obscure the reality that the entire colonial project itself was a misguided and racist machine; hence, the historian ought to extract and interpret carefully information with these caveats and inherent biases in mind.[54] That there were, in fact, kindhearted colonists and fair-minded colonial policy makers who fervently wanted to extend the tenets of universal republicanism to the colonies does not erase the psychological and material fallout of colonial interventionism.[55] Moreover, it is not my specific intention to either indict or absolve any individual actor for his or her role in the colonial project; rather, I intend to try to understand why rational actors holding diverse views and understandings chose, were coerced, silently complied, or rejected at their peril sundry schemes of the mission to civilize or regenerate.

It is my intention to eschew the excessively common mistake of reducing the histories of science and medicine to an encomium of advances conceived without conflict in a sociopolitical vacuum. Although science operates under the guise of objectivity and neutrality, it is the social, cultural, and political push and pull that make science itself a variable and provoked the ambiguity of decision makers, both in France and in Tunisia, that are described in this book. Even when scientists and physicians, regardless of their national origin or religious affiliation, accept the same codes of conduct—the same criteria for the reception of evidentiary value, testing protocols, and the elaboration of results—differences remain. With appeals to the detached reason of science and medicine, colonial projects claimed purity and objectivity, but the expansion of so-called Western science and medicine was in fact a normative (and normalizing) mission, often tainted by bogus racial science, faulty medical assumptions, bourgeois socioeconomic interests, and political imperatives. Colonial administrators and protectorate authorities tried valiantly to mask cleverly or steer clear of ideologically driven policies, but they did not hesitate to call on the *science* of regeneration, which, although manipulated by political and social forces, purportedly transcended ideological influence.[56] According to this vein of thought, political and social ideologies may be the overly chatty handmaidens of scientific and medical authority, but they possess no inherent power of their own, aside from the rhetorical. In contrast, science and medicine gain their authority from an appeal to empiricism, objective analysis, and rigorous examination of competing hypotheses. Without scientific and medical authority, political and social ideologies can convince and cajole, but they cannot plausibly make substantive claims of "truth." Of course, the reality is that more than we care to admit, science and medicine are the result of a complex array of social, political, and cultural processes that inform and influence our hypotheses, expectations, and even our "objective" analyses.[57]

To capture the inner workings of a discrete community and to explore more deeply the warp and weft of the rhetorical power of regeneration and its attendant results, this book utilizes the methodological framework of the social and cultural history of medicine augmented by microhistorical accounts. Microhistories and archival narratives, when compared to and buttressed by the broader historical record, disclose a tale more rich and more complex than a mere recitation of an overarching historical catalogue of data pertaining to Jewish life in the Maghrib. History often privileges the narratives that recall the transmission of scientific knowledge to the hapless colonial dependent or the construction and installation of modern conveniences in the midst of "native disorder" but ignore entirely the ways in which indigenous communities understood, absorbed, reinterpreted, or even rejected these "facts" and "modernities." For example, it is an important historical fact, clearly documented in the French archives, that the protectorate invested heavily in residential infrastructure in the Jewish quarter of Tunis and offered new apartments fitted with modern, private kitchens within each unit. However, it is perhaps more important to appreciate how Jewish women, accustomed to sharing a brazier in an open courtyard with ten other women, understood and reacted to this adaptation to modernity. Nonetheless, a reliance on local microhistory does not dictate that the cultural historian be tied to an overly schematic *Annalistes* approach, which, unfortunately—and I think unintentionally—tends to minimize the agency and influence of individual actors on the broad scope of history.[58] The local and microhistorical analyses detailed in this short book are not intended as an all-purpose, totalizing portrayal of "life as a French colonial subject"; however, these analyses do provide powerful illustrations of how rational actors within a community, often under great stress, used the tools at their disposal to construct and understand their place in a newly emerging social and political order.[59]

Although I remain cognizant of the limitations of an excessively localized approach, there do exist isolated and perhaps even anomalous historical happenings that occurred within the broad community, among the myriad demographic voices of women, children, Jews, Christians, Muslims, and metropolitan and colonial elites, as well as among those in the Jewish ghetto, that individually mean little but when gathered together express a unique tale in their entirety. Like the dots and smudges of an Impressionist painting, which only make intellectual sense when viewed as a totality and from a removed perspective, the vignettes of microhistory, when woven into the broader historical narrative, can create a unique historical tableau. Sometimes there are histories that are so localized, so particular to a group of people, a place, and a time, that we wonder what we, as historians, could possibly glean from an analysis of such accounts. It is true that the dots and smudges—the argument in the market, the act of defying a colonial official, the contested soccer match—mean little in the abstract but, when reconstructed and reintegrated into the framework of a broader narrative, take on the fresh and complex meanings that make up the vivid tapestry of life.[60]

Chapter 2 of this book describes the creation of "modern space" in colonial Tunis. It recounts the foundation of the municipal sanitary infrastructure and outlines the efforts undertaken by French authorities to harness the powerful rhetoric of both sanitary science and laboratory-based medical authority to create a system of bureaucracies and legal ordinances that could be used to redraw the map of Tunis. This chapter also considers contemporary French notions of race, class, and "belonging" and the way these ideas reshaped the spatial organization of the city of Tunis. French colonial urban planning in Tunis demonstrates the concerted efforts of the regime to segregate the populace not just along the "traditional" lines of colonizer/colonized but also according to religious confession and socio-economic milieu. In efforts similar to early twentieth-century racial zoning in the United States, colonial authorities implemented strict guidelines to separate the "races," religions, and classes of Tunis.

Chapter 3 depicts the complex history surrounding the decision to destroy (i.e., "modernize") the hara of Tunis. It describes how elites in both Paris and Tunis attempted to completely remake Tunisian Jewish society and space according to a totalizing utopian vision.[61] It also exposes the doublespeak of colonial officials who recast destruction as the "start of the tortuous inevitable road to development and modernization," a process that ultimately bifurcated space in Tunis into exotic, "Arab" enclaves and historically uniform, modern "French" *quartiers*.[62]

Through a comparative analysis of the hygienic debates in Paris and Tunis at the beginning of the twentieth century, this chapter describes how progressive policies that had been abandoned in the metropole were actively and aggressively pursued in the colonies and explores the justifications for these dramatic differences in the implementation of municipal urban renewal policy, along with the various interests that attempted to influence the debate. This discussion dispels the mythology of an "aseptic and self-generating Europe, historically formed without any contact with other cultures."[63]

Chapter 4 discusses the quest for the modern, regenerated Tunisian Jewish mind and body and the struggle over who would be the architect of this social, cultural, and corporeal transformation: the conservative, "civilizing" forces of the AIU, backed by the power of the colonial regime, or the vibrant voice of Zionism, bolstered by Jewish pride and muscular strength? This chapter centers on the competing modernities that battled for the hearts and minds of Tunis's Jews, especially its youth, and describes the epistemic fissures and concrete differences that developed between

Zionism and the AIU, both of which perceived of and presented themselves to the Tunisian Jewish public as pillars of "modernity" and "social hygiene."

This chapter presents a history of the efforts to regenerate a community, which is a concept so indelibly linked to the personal and corporeal nature of science and medicine that it is particularly well suited for the highly subjective accounts so often associated with microhistory. Stories and descriptions that so heavily impinge on the intimacies of the human body, its fragilities and failings and its triumphs and strengths, are fertile ground for the sociocultural historian of medicine wishing to reconstruct and reimagine the inner workings of both the conceptual and material expressions of regeneration.

Chapter 5 of this book challenges notions of patriarchal supremacy and the power of modern science and medicine over women's health. Counter to the metanarrative of "saving babies" with modern science, in this chapter I attribute the reduced infant mortality in the Tunisian Jewish community of the interwar years to the intervention of Tunisian Jewish women rather than to modern "men's science." Jewish women in Tunis not only successfully negotiated a seat at the table as "Western biomedicine" sought to relocate childbirth from female-centered homebirth to male-centered hospital birth; they also formed powerful "homemaker networks" independent from male authority. Within the confines of these networks, Tunisian Jewish women elaborated their own definitions of science, modern femininity, motherhood, and medicine.

Taken as a whole, this book describes the ideological, scientific, and cultural exchanges between the metropole and the Tunisian Jewish community and the way the community influenced, changed, and reinterpreted the messages of regeneration and modernity in unforeseen ways. Just as the secular Third Republic, in an ironic twist, used Catholic missionaries as an economically effective way to spread France's civilizing mission and fulfill its promises of Republican universal equality in colonial space, the Jewish community also harnessed the strength and resources of its faithful to spread the message of regeneration in the Maghrib.[64] Anticlericalism, which pitted secular administrators and missionaries into pitched battles for the "hearts and minds" of their colonial subjects, cast constant scrutiny on the Church's motives, and limited its intellectual mobility, was not an impediment for the Jewish community. Although there were rifts and divides within the Jewish community, Jews from outside Tunisia—and differing factions within Tunisia—regularly used Judaism as a network of similarly situated individuals through which to spread their particular brand of regeneration.

Examinations of French colonialism in the Maghrib must consider more deeply the meanings and significance of analytical constructs such as race, religion, ethnicity, and nationality by reinterpreting and redefining the "flattening rubric of identity."[65] On the surface, this may appear to be a semantic argument; however, reappraising our understanding of identity as a continuous process of competing discourses shows that identity is unstable, ever changing, and disjointed. Woven throughout this book are lively examples of the overlapping and often contradictory discourses that constructed unique identities, like the Tunisian Jewish colonial identity, and in turn shaped social and political action in both the metropole and Tunisia. A reexamination of these multifaceted discourses shows that understandings of the regenerated self, viewed in social, cultural, political, and existential terms, flowed back and forth across the Mediterranean and reached an apex during the interwar years (1919–39).

The Janus face of regeneration—degeneration—was a tidy metaphor that was elastic enough to encapsulate every conceivable threat: physical weakness, moral turpitude, urban blight, unruly children, and uppity women. All of these problems had logical explanations and rational solutions grounded in science. The positivism of science in the nineteenth and early twentieth centuries presented itself as a comprehensive antidote—universally applicable and rooted in objectivity. Science and its ability to effect the wholesale regeneration of entire populations validated and buttressed the widely divergent social and political ideologies of the age, like Saint-Simonianism, expansionist colonialism, French Republicanism, and Zionism. Even when positivism faced philosophical challenges in the early twentieth century, scientific and medical authority remained strong enough to justify a sustained belief in the validity of mutable biological determinism and its related promise of regeneration, at least in the colonial context.

Despite its apparent advantages for Maghribi Jews, the narrative of willing adaptation to French colonization, especially when recounted through the lens of the regenerationist crusade, does run the risk of oversimplifying and leveling the arc of history. The power of scientific and medical authority was monumental, and the messages of regeneration that this authority promoted were difficult to ignore; however, the *responses* to the messages of regeneration were far from preordained. In fact, this book describes myriad ways in which the message was accepted, reinterpreted, ignored, or used at cross-purpose. Regeneration was not a catalyst to inevitable modernization; it was a medically justified, scientifically based theory that shaped political, social, and cultural ideologies in unforeseen and often counterintuitive ways.

2 Regenerating Space

Destruction and Divided Communities

Do not become a stranger to yourself, for you are lost from that day on; you will have no peace if there is not, somewhere within you, a corner of certainty, calm waters where you can take refuge in sleep.

— ALBERT MEMMI, *The Colonizer and the Colonized*

The most dramatic effects of the regeneration movement can be seen in the ways in which the French regime imbibed the messages that connected "race," class, environment, and potential moral and physical fitness. This chapter describes how, over the course of several decades of French rule, Tunis was radically transformed from a diverse city in which residents of various identity groups freely and, for the most part, peacefully shared space into a city that was Balkanized into ethnic, religious, and class-based enclaves. The protectorate, using the new tools of public health and hygiene, implemented myriad regulations that scrutinized the salubriousness of the urban environment for the city's inhabitants. However, these regulations were not evenly applied. In fact, for reasons that this chapter will elucidate, the protectorate determined that areas linked to French and Jewish interests, such the new French quarter (*ville nouvelle*), La Goulette (a seaside Tunis suburb), and the hara, required massive intervention and even destruction in the path to re-creation, whereas predominately Muslim areas of Tunis, or at least areas associated with Muslims, like the Kasbah and the souks of the medina, were worthy of "preservation" and a laissez-faire attitude in regard to the enforcement of sanitary regulations. As a result, the ideas and actions that linked "regenerated" space and intrusive governmental oversight with "Frenchness" and potential "fitness" became firmly rooted in the consciousness of an entire generation of metropolitan *tunisois*. The effects of this linkage will be seen in this and subsequent chapters.

French involvement in, and eventual colonization of, North Africa followed a spasmodic trajectory and was for the most part poorly planned and rather ill conceived. The failing regime of Charles X invaded Algeria in 1830 and ensuing regimes — monarchical, imperial, and republican — desperate to show military strength vis-à-vis Great Britain or to divert the attention of voters away from government ineptitude in metropolitan France, colonized and subsequently incorporated Algeria into France as three *départements* in 1848.[1] Jews in these areas of Algeria were naturalized en masse in 1870.[2]

In neighboring Tunisia, the European powers increasingly challenged the hegemony of the ruling Husaynid dynasty and forced the bey, Muhammad al-Sadiq (reign 1859–81), to make a series of economic and political concessions. In September 1857 French gunboat diplomacy forced Muhammad al-Sadiq's predecessor, Muhammad Bey (reign 1855–1859), to issue the Fundamental Pact (Ar. ʿAhd al-Amān). Under this edict, all of the bey's subjects were guaranteed security regardless of race, nationality, or religion. Jews were liberated from many of the legal disabilities of *dhimmi* status and other discriminatory regulations, such as dress codes, corvée, and confinement in the Jewish quarter, the hara. There is academic debate as to how strictly the rule to confine Jews to the hara was actually enforced; even before the Fundamental Pact, there were wealthy Jews who lived on the outskirts of the hara and in the northern suburbs of Tunis.

By the mid-nineteenth century, Tunisia was heavily in debt to several of the Western powers, and its ability to make good on its obligations was very much in doubt. For the vast majority of Tunisian Jews, both

Twansa and Grana, economic hardship was a fact of life.[3] France, Great Britain, and Italy all sought to take advantage of this economic weakness to increase their influence in Tunisia. At the Congress of Berlin in 1878, in a move to limit the power of the Ottoman Empire, the Western Powers partitioned the Balkans, recognized British control of Egypt and Cyprus, and gave France free rein in Tunisia. Although illustrative of the chessboard mentality taken by Europeans, especially in regard to areas south of the Mediterranean Sea, ceding Cyprus to Great Britain was merely the tip of the iceberg in the various concessions involved in the Scramble for Africa. Between 1878 and World War I, the entire continent, save Liberia and Ethiopia, was ruthlessly subjugated to European imperial domination. For the most part, the Maghrib fell under French control, except for Italian expansion into Tripolitania and Spanish claims on portions of Morocco. In spite of Italy's political and diplomatic blundering, Italians in Tunisia continued to outnumber the French until the eve of World War II and played an important role in French political machinations.

After the invasion of Algeria by French troops in 1830, France reorganized Algeria, save stretches of the Saharan south, into French departments, which were annexed to mainland France in 1848. Because of different sociopolitical conditions, such as colonial tensions with Italy and Great Britain and the aftermath of the defeat in the Franco-Prussian War, the French could not overtly exert such a heavy hand in Tunisia. Predicated on an "incursion" by a Tunisian tribe into Franco-Algerian territory, French troops invaded Tunisia in 1881 and forced Muhammad Bey to sign the Treaty of Bardo (May 12, 1881), giving France control over Tunisian foreign affairs. In exchange for the refinancing of Tunisia's debts by the French government, combined with gunboat diplomacy and the invasion of thirty-six thousand French expeditionary troops, Muhammad Bey's successor, Ali Bey (reign 1882–1902), signed the La Marsa Convention on June 8, 1883, which transferred full domestic administrative control to a French resident general and established Tunisia as a French protectorate.[4] Under the legal fiction of the protectorate, the bey remained as titular head of state but little else. From this point forward, all power in Tunisia was vested primarily in the resident general who assumed the role of "prime minister, comptroller of the country's finances, and commander of its armed forces."[5] Various French officials filled the interstices of power that the protectorate had not reserved as the exclusive domain of the resident general. For all intents and purposes, the power of the bey was reduced to a rubber stamp.

From the installation of the French regime in Tunisia in 1881, the French hold over the Tunisian people was tenuous. According to Resident General Lucien Saint, Italian claims on Tunisia (where Italians outnumbered the French until the 1930s) and the emergence of indigenous nationalist movements, such as the Destour Party, were the two most palpable obstacles to peaceful domination over Tunisia. To combat these impediments, Saint and the subsequent administration of François Manceron bolstered the number of French citizens in relation to Italians by accepting (and counting in the censes) select Tunisian Jews as "French" and countered nationalist movements by marginalizing Muslims and driving a wedge between Jews and Muslims.[6] In an era of tentative rapprochement between Jews and Muslims, French officials pursued a strict segregationist housing policy that separated Tunisians according to religion, "race," and class.

This strategy of Balkanizing the indigenous people, peeling away Tunisian Jews through "special treatment" and naturalization, and isolating Muslims into "authentic" Oriental enclaves provided an expedient neutralization to what France perceived as obstacles to supremacy in Tunisia: Italian threats from without and indigenous national threats from within. To advance their aims, the French relied on the unlikely but highly modern tools of public health and urban reform. The French protectorate's concern for the health and well-being of Tunisia's people—indigenous and settlers alike—offered a benign pretext for distinct divide-and-conquer strategies that the latest theories of public health and urban reformation justified. These strategies permitted the French to parcel the population of Tunis into discrete enclaves according to religious and class distinctions.

To recapitulate, through an examination of public health ordinances in Tunis and the neighboring commune of La Goulette, an area with a high Jewish, Italian, and Maltese population, this chapter demonstrates that colonial authorities pursued two radically divergent strategies regarding the enforcement of hygienic reforms. The default policy, which was universally applied in Jewish and non-Muslim areas, like La Goulette, the hara, and the French *ville nouvelle*, was modernization by way of highly intrusive regulation or destruction.[7] On the other hand, areas with "Oriental authenticity," such as the Muslim areas of the medina, were to be preserved and exempted from regulation.

The Structure of the Protectorate Regime

For administrative purposes, the French divided Tunisia into five regions (*provinces*)—Tunis, Bizerte, Kef, Sousse, and Sfax—which were administered by French regional chiefs. Each region was subdivided into nineteen districts (*communes*), each overseen by a French civil controller (*contrôleur civil*).[8] To quell dissent and preserve the guise of Tunisian control of internal affairs, the civil controllers maintained the local power of the *qadāt* (Ar., sing., *qāʿid*) in the cities and *shuyukh* (Ar., sing., *shaykh*) in the countryside for the direct administration of beylical decrees and the collection of taxes.[9] Fifty-nine municipalities, including Tunis and its entry port, La Goulette, were granted special status that allowed them to form municipal councils (*conseils municipaux*) to regulate urban affairs.

French settler (*colon*) interests dominated all representative and deliberative bodies under the protectorate regime. In 1892 the protectorate, under the tutelage of Resident General Justin Massicault, organized the Consultative Conference (Conférence Consultative), which had no official power and served simply as a venue for French settlers to air their grievances. Indigenous Tunisians had no voice at all until 1907, when sixteen Tunisians were added to the conference. Under protest from French *colons* that "natives" possessed too much power under the new structure, the protectorate revised the system and divided the conference into three sections: one for Tunisians, who were appointed by the French, and two for French. The attempt to suppress increased indigenous political representation met widespread protest and forced the protectorate to scrap the conference altogether.

The Grand Council of Tunisia (Grand Conseil de Tunisie), formed by the Saint regime in 1922, replaced the Consultative Conference but in reality initiated very few democratic changes. The council was a bicameral body with a French section of fifty-two members elected by direct vote and a "native section" of twenty-six members elected by the vote of "indigenous notables" handpicked by the regime.[10] One member of the native section was a Jew chosen by the elders of the Jewish community. Although the regime allotted slightly more decision-making authority to the council than it had to the conference, the council remained egregiously tipped in favor of French settler opinion. In the unlikely event that indigenous voices could rally enough support to carry a proposal, the resident general held an ace up his sleeve: absolute veto power.[11] Most residents general ruled Tunisia as a fiefdom with relatively little oversight or direct intervention from metropolitan France. Unlike in Algeria, the early residents general of Tunisia were adamant that the French military would play no administrative role in the regional governments of Tunisia.[12]

The oversight of public health and hygiene in Tunisia during the colonial era (1881–1956) operated on three distinct bureaucratic levels: the municipal, the communal (regional), and the national. The Tunis Sanitary Council, established by Mustafa Bey in 1835, was the first European-run agency in Tunisia, albeit one reserved for an advisory role.[13] In 1885 the colonial regime took direct control of the oversight of hygiene and sanitation by appropriating the governance of the Sanitary Council and strengthening its administrative powers and enforcement mechanisms. The primary goal of the protectorate's Sanitary Council—comprising two Tunis municipal councilmen, two representatives from the Chamber of Commerce, and two physicians—was to monitor ships arriving at La Goulette for signs of infection and to oversee Tunis's three lazarettos (plague hospitals).[14] Over the several decades following the establishment of the 1885 iteration of the Sanitary Council, the responsibility for hygiene and sanitation passed from the auspices of the secretary general in 1897 to a newly created Office of Public Assistance in the Department of the Interior in 1911. In 1920 the protectorate added additional layers to the national bureaucracy: the Office of Public Assistance was renamed the Directorate of Hygiene, led by the formidable bacteriologist Etienne Burnet, and subdivided into offices that dealt with public hygiene, maritime health, and public assistance.[15] During the interwar years, the divisions and subdivisions of offices, bureaus, and directorates became more and more byzantine. In 1928 the Service for Assistance and Public Hygiene (SAPH) supplanted the Directorate of Hygiene. The SAPH, under the auspices of the Department of the Interior, was responsible for overall public assistance, public and maritime hygiene, social hygiene, and the supervision of doctors and hospitals that provided assistance. But the new SAPH shared overlapping administrative purview with the Service for Regional and Communal Administration (SRCA). The SRCA was responsible for overseeing the regional administration of hygiene and health and the communal administration of doctors and hospitals. In essence, the SAPH and the SRCA sought the same ends, yet competed for authority and funding.

The knotted national bureaucracy was further aggravated in 1930, when Resident General François Manceron created the autonomous Office of Social Hygiene and Preventative Medicine, which competed with the two preexisting health and hygiene services (SAPH and SRCA) for the authority to control national health care. French representatives—steeped in the political ideology of the Third Republic—advocated over-bureaucratization and promoted a pathological fear of consolidated centralized power, which resulted in a dilution of the national public health infrastructure in Tunisia to a point of confusion that rendered it inoperable. The situation was ameliorated in 1937, when Resident General Armand Guillon decreed that all services that dealt with public health, hygiene, public assistance, and sanitation in Tunisia would be regrouped under the Directorate of Public Health and Assistance, which would report directly to the secretary general of the Tunisian government (as had been the case from 1897 to 1911). In short, the oversight of public health at the national level in Tunisia was confused at best. Although the new directorate finally had the authority to pass reform measures at the national level, the communes and municipalities—many of which had existed for several decades by this point—were already accustomed to wielding what little authority they possessed to enact their own reforms. Regardless of whether the impetus for structural public health reform emanated from the national or local level, it was the French who exercised political control and held the purse strings. However, French authorities recognized that the promulgation of extensive and invasive reforms proved far more manageable when issued from and overseen at the local level. Tunis and La Goulette were two localities that used their newfound powers to enact sweeping public health, urban planning, and infrastructural reforms.[16] The repudiation of filth and disorder evidenced the driving desire of local municipal officials together with representatives of the protectorate regime to embrace normative, bourgeois notions of individual and collective cleanliness in the quest for modernity.[17]

The municipality of Tunis was reorganized by the protectorate in 1883 and paralleled the creation of the neighboring commune of La Goulette in 1884. Tunis and La Goulette occupied the west and the east banks of Lake Tunis respectively, with La Goulette serving as the only channel of entry into the lake and as the port of Tunis. La Goulette, because of its seaport, had long been considered an entry point for various diseases that ravaged Tunisia. In 1908 the protectorate created the Tunis Office of Municipal Hygiene to combat repeated epidemics of cholera, typhus, and typhoid that devastated indigenous populations. The local offices of hygiene in both Tunis and La Goulette possessed wide-reaching authority to regulate private and public thoroughfares, housing structures, and food preparation, as well as vaccination and disinfection. The localities also dictated in what areas new sewer lines would be laid and controlled the distribution of running water. These broad powers over public health ordinances and urban planning proved to be the perfect tools to redraw the map of Tunis and its suburbs.[18]

Sewers and Water Supply

In 1883 the renowned laboratory researcher and physician Robert Koch paid a visit to North Africa as the head of the German Cholera Commission to investigate yet another outbreak of the disease that had been the scourge of the nineteenth century. While in North Africa, Koch identified and isolated for the first time the bacterial agent responsible for the deaths of millions: *Vibrio cholerae*. Although the etiology of cholera and its mode of transmission had long been suspected, thanks in large part to the work of British physician and "father of epidemiology" John Snow, the "pure samples" of the bacteria that Koch carried back to Germany as the subject of further research definitively confirmed what had long been suspected: cholera was a specific disease transmitted as a result of poor sewage facilities and unclean drinking water.

As a result of Koch's research, French hygienists, who had already begun the crusade for sewage systems in the metropole, redoubled their focus on urban renewal. Under the Third Republic, Paris, "in terms of size and scope, its place in the nation and imperial self-conception, and its relation to the massive industrialization earlier in the century," was the primary focus of these efforts.[19] But pushed by the zeal of their mission to civilize, these experts voiced concern for the colonies as well. Colonists were in heightened danger of infection, as according to the latest medical knowledge, "parasites and germs are spread three ways: water, small animals, and indigenous people."[20] But just as in France, expense and logistics necessitated the rationing of large-scale infrastructural development. Starting with a modest budget, the Institut Pasteur de Tunis, under the direction of Adrien Loir, who was assisted by Nobel Prize winner Charles Nicolle, focused primarily on curtailing the scourge of epidemic disease.[21] The protectorate regime realized that careful investment in the colonial medical infrastructure could appease indigenous interests and boost the prestige of the regime.

During the early years of the French protectorate, before the hygienists concerned themselves with Tunisia, the urban inhabitants of Tunis improvised the management of raw sewage collected in septic pits. A septic pit is not to be confused with a septic system. A septic pit, or cesspit, is not designed to "weep" or leech back into the environment any water that is separated from sewage. Instead, it is simply a holding tank that must be emptied on a regular basis. However, in lieu of having tanks emptied, when the pits began to overflow, residents dug trenches connecting the dwelling's cesspit to the nearest principal street. Principal streets—which were pitched inward, hence highest at the curb—had a trough dug down the center that received the flow of sewage and wastewater. This black water, washed along by rainwater during the rainy season, flowed down the center of the principal streets to open air trenches called *khandaqat* (Ar., sing., *khandaq*). Following the natural slope of the land (from the heights of the Kasbah, through the medina, toward the mostly unoccupied lowlands at the lakeshore), the *khandaqat* emptied into Lake Tunis. The public health consequences of such a system, especially for those at the lowest elevations of the medina (the Jewish hara), are evident.

Although the municipality of Tunis installed 132 kilometers of sewer pipes between 1891 and the beginning of World War I, most of this was slated for the rectilinear streets of the *ville nouvelle*, which stretched from the eastern edge of the medina through the lowlands skirting the western shore of Lake Tunis.[22] In a similar fashion, the seaside suburb of La Goulette laid sewer pipe apace, but only those residents whose dwellings faced onto a street containing a sewer line (invariably one of the "modern" rectilinear streets) were required to connect. For those who lived in areas equipped with sewer lines, strict regulations required any previously existing homeowners and landlords to connect their property to the sewer line within six months of service becoming available.[23] In addition, all existing septic tanks and *khandaqat*, whether in use or not, had to be cleansed and filled within this six-month period.[24] However, according to municipal officials, the narrow, twisted streets of the "Arab" medina precluded the feasibility of sewer installation and continued in the use of *fossé d'aisance*, or septic pits.

Even outside the medina, septic pits remained the norm in houses that did not face onto a street with a sewer, albeit with significantly more stringent regulation by local authorities. Communal authorities required that pits be emptied (*vidange des fossés*) and disinfected on a regular basis, but only after seeking approval and oversight by community health officials. Landowners had to prove to authorities that they possessed the necessary equipment and disinfectant required to complete the task. During the emptying operation, public health officials meticulously monitored for leakage of gaseous vapors, equipped workers lowered into the pits with safety harnesses, and placed lanterns on the streets that warned passersby of the noxious activities taking place.[25] Extraction of waste was permitted from the first of October to the end of March, between 10:00 p.m. and

5:00 a.m., and from the first of April to end of September, between 11:00 p.m. and 6:00 a.m. All extracted waste was emptied into municipal-owned septic tanks located at least five hundred meters from any habitation and covered with disinfectant.[26] The commune reserved the right to clean and disinfect without delay—at the expense of the landowner—any septic pit viewed as a public health menace. Again, these sanitary measures were not implemented in the Kasbah and the "Arab" medina.

In many ways, the quest for clean drinking water was even more contentious than the proper disposal of wastewater and more clearly demonstrates the arbitrary, heavy hand of colonial authority vis-à-vis public opinion and indigenous leaders. Although wells were permitted to private landowners (with a multitude of regulations, including regular inspection), local ordinances required that all landlords of multifamily buildings and restaurants hold a subscription to the water company (*l'eau de Zaghouan*).[27] *L'eau de Zaghouan* refers to water provided by an ancient Roman aqueduct built in the second century CE. Believed to be the second longest Roman aqueduct ever built, the Zaghouan aqueduct, which carries water 57.5 miles (92.5 kilometers) from the Tunisian interior highlands to the Tunisian coast, was restored by French architects in the mid-nineteenth century but remained in the hands of a Tunisian-owned water company. In 1884 the Directorate of Public Works, sanctioned by the majority of the Tunis Municipal Council, "transferred" ownership of the Zaghouan water company to the French-owned, Paris-based water company Durand et Cie. The new management in turn pushed the Municipal Council to mandate the installation of meters to measure water usage and, of course, to levy a consumption tax. In spite of the hue and cry provoked by the company's seizure of the water supply of greater Tunis and the increase in the cost of water, the protectorate refused to cede control of the vital commodity back into indigenous hands.[28] Compounding anger over the increased regulation and price of water, new ordinances mandated that traditional indigenous structures, such as *funduqs* and *wakālas*, use *l'eau de Zaghouan*.[29] Before the twentieth century, a *funduq* described a "neutral" commercial space where Muslims, Jews, and Christians gathered to trade goods on parcels of land conceded by the Ottoman Empire. *Funduqs* usually provided sleeping quarters for the visiting merchants and were often named for the nationality of the merchants who frequented them, that is, *funduq des Anglais*, *funduq des Italiens*, and so forth.[30] A *wakāla* is a building that is divided and often further subdivided into a large number of living spaces (a cross between a tenement and a boarding house). In the early twentieth century, as the population of Tunis and the surrounding areas exploded, *funduqs* and *wakālas* became increasingly overcrowded housing of last resort for the poorest of the poor. The owners of these densely populated urban structures, now subjected to paying for metered water to ensure the health of their residents, were stretched to their financial limits. During the early twentieth century, the increased scrutiny by colonial officials of indigenous homes and the regulation of hitherto personal sanitation practices had become not only normative but also, in select areas, codified into law. As indigenous property owners fell behind in their struggles to fulfill the demands of French regulations, the capability of Tunisians to bear the burden and responsibilities of property ownership was called into question by French authorities. Property owners who would not or could not comply with burdensome and expensive hygienic regulations further justified French calls for "intervention" on a grander scale.

Mal aria, "Bad Air"

Contemporary descriptions of urban life in the nineteenth century, whether recording events in Paris, Bombay, London, or Tunis, are remarkably uniform on several concerns: filth, squalor, and disease were omnipresent facets of the urban condition. In the first half of the nineteenth century, scientists and physicians explained the link between filth and disease through the miasmatic theory. Before the elaboration of the germ theory in the 1870s, which identified precise microscopic agents as causative of specific diseases, scientists and physicians blamed illness on the miasmatic emanations from organic putrefaction, inadequately drained soil, and poorly washed bodies. According to the miasmatic theory, low-lying, poorly ventilated areas and those that were overcrowded were prone to the development of fermentations that deleteriously altered the quality of the air. Exposure to the miasmas emanating from these regions of "bad air" (*mal aria*) provoked imbalances in the body that could cause both chronic and acute illnesses. Exposure to exciting factors, such as hypersexuality, intemperance, or vicious behavior, made an individual even more susceptible to the ill effects of noxious miasmas, thus introducing an awkward element of blame and shame into disease diagnosis. But in spite of the paradigmatic shift in scientific belief in regard to disease etiology from a theory that was environmental and miasmatic to one that was highly particularized and based on microscopic entities, the underlying issue in the eyes of the public when thinking of disease and disorder remained the same: filth, dirt, and stench, coupled with some element of misbehavior, caused disease.[31]

The myriad regulations regarding sewage and water supply demonstrate that hygienic experts in Tunis, such as Charles Nicolle, Ernest Conseil, and Adrien Loir, understood the etiology and modes of transmission for killers, such as cholera and other enteric diseases; however, the debunked miasmatic theory of disease etiology was hard to shake. Although scientists articulated the germ theory of disease etiology during the 1870s, public health officials continued their obsessive focus on miasmatic theory and the attendant preventive and curative effects of fresh air and sunlight. As a result, in spite of the massive efforts exercised by public health officials to install sewers, mandate the proper function and usage of toilet facilities, and regulate the water supply, many officials expressed far more concern regarding the availability of fresh air and sunlight.[32]

Of course, there was nothing new in the idea that "bad air" caused disease. Dating back to the Hippocratic texts, physicians and empirics alike had lauded the beneficial effects of sunshine and fresh air. According to French hygienists, adhering to the miasmatic theory in spite of counter-evidence was not meant to ignore "germs," but it did lend credence to the idea that a particular area or space can represent an "overall nuisance" to the community.[33]

In keeping with the theory that an abundance of green plants and trees would rid the surrounding environment of "the fermenting particles and odors that the Ancients called miasmas," colonial officials advocated the introduction of green space in Tunis and the implementation of practices that would increase the penetration of air and sunlight. To this end, the city gardener of Paris presented his final plans for Tunis's Parc du Belvédère in 1892.[34] This vast 110 hectare plot of land—a former olive grove—situated on the top of a hill overlooking Tunis from the north was laid out as an "English-style" garden characterized by open lawns dotted with groves of trees and flower beds. The park provided an urban retreat from the heat of the city during the oppressive summer heat waves. However, to French officials, the park was not finished without an embellishment that would introduce a vibrant, Oriental flare to the cool, wooded European expanse. In 1910 officials successfully moved and restored a dilapidated pavilion—the *Koubba al-Haoua*—from a palace in neighboring Manouba to the peak of the highest hill in the park. The original purpose of the *Koubba*—to commemorate the site of a holy shrine—was irrelevant to colonial officials, who viewed it merely as a random expression of Oriental architecture. The new park, crowned by its *Koubba*, opened to great fanfare in 1910. Although city officials claimed that the *Koubba* was placed in the park to please indigenous Muslims, it was more likely put there, much like the mocked-up souks of the Colonial Exposition in Paris, to satisfy the Western desire to live and experience the Orient within the comfort of planned European space. In any case, colonial officials stressed that the park provided fresh air and a respite from the crowded city.

Neighboring La Goulette, however, had no Parc du Belvédère to provide its residents with the salubrious "oxidation" provided by planned green space. Situated on a narrow isthmus of land between the Mediterranean Sea and the murky Lake Tunis, strict regulation governing the dimensions of habitable interior space in relation to availability of fresh air was the only viable alternative for La Goulette to ensure proper "oxidation" of living quarters. For example, according to hygienists, each adult required 18 cubic meters of air to breath easily; children required 12 cubic meters each. Therefore, a room that was 3 meters long, 4 meters deep, and 3 meters high (36 cubic meters) could accommodate two adults or three children under the age of fifteen. Hence, if the ceiling height was expanded, the number of occupants could be as well. For this room of 36 square meters, a window of 1.8 square meters was required—the windows' dimensions depended on the overall dimensions of the room, which were in turn based on a sufficient amount of cubic air available to each inhabitant.[35]

To comply with the new recommendations, the community of La Goulette mandated that every room, whether inhabited by day or by night, had to measure at least 20 cubic meters and that every sleeping space had to allow at least 11 cubic meters per person. Although the La Goulette mandates fell short of the French recommendations for cubic meters per person, the regulations compensated by allocating more square meters to window size. According to city code, ground floor windows had to be at least 2 square meters and upper floor windows 1.5 square meters per 20 cubic meters of interior space—every additional 30 cubic meters of interior space required an additional square meter of window space.[36] All windows had to have direct access to the street or courtyard, and *jours de souffrance* (windows that permit light but cannot be opened) were not legally counted as windows.[37]

Urban planners, inspired by French hygienist Albert Besson's ideas of "*l'hygiène de l'habitation*," began to articulate a vision for structures, infrastructures, and neighborhoods that would be built or razed and rebuilt in "non-historical" areas of Tunis.[38] Initial regulation dating from 1899 required that building height in Tunis could not exceed 11.6 meters on streets that were six to eight meters wide, 18.6 meters for streets eight to ten meters wide, and 20 meters for streets more than 10 meters wide. Zones identified as historical, such as large parts of the Kasbah and medina, where most streets were three to five meters wide and were often crisscrossed by elevated passages between the upper floors of buildings, were exempt from regulation. The regulations were further amended to *require* that the height of newly constructed buildings meet *specific* height requirements based on the vertical height of the construction in relation to the edifices on the opposite side of the street. This decree ensured the absolute uniformity of building heights on newly constructed streets and avenues in the *ville nouvelle*.[39] In addition to symmetrical uniformity, regulated building height ensured that those at street level would enjoy a pleasing orderly view and have access to the holy grail of hygienic requirements: sunlight and fresh air. Besson stressed the links among substandard housing, lack of sunlight, and epidemic disease, primarily tuberculosis.[40]

Hygienists asserted that cleaning and whitewashing the exterior of buildings and courtyards was paramount to maintaining health in crowded city streets. Alleyways, stairwells, and hallways used by the public had to be cleansed and whitewashed every year.[41] By whitening the exterior walls, the sun's solar rays would be more readily reflected and light diffused onto the streets. Health officials mandated that "open windows were a daily necessity, not only for fresh air, but for the anti-septic qualities of the sunlight."[42] The cleansing rays of the sun could spread all over through reflection and diffusion, even on winter days when the sun's slant is low on the horizon. Although most of the indigenously built structures in Tunis were whitewashed, they lacked the required exterior spatial layout required to reap the maximum benefits of the sun's cleansing rays. French health authorities posited that even on "December 21, the shortest day of the year when the sun's rays are at their most oblique, the foundation of *every* building must be illuminated by the sun *for an hour*."[43] To achieve this goal, urban planners and hygienists suggested a north-south orientation of residential streets. Furthermore, the width of the streets had to be adjusted according to the height of the buildings occupying said street. For example, a one-story building required a street at least 8 meters wide, whereas the typical apartment buildings (between three and five stories) required street widths of 15 to 21 meters to ensure that the sun's cleansing rays could penetrate to the street surface. The requirements for east-west streets were even more stringent. Every 15 meters of street-front height required a width of 10 meters for a north-south road and 15 meters for an east-west road. "For streets that are oriented east-west, where one of the sides is nearly always deprived of the sun, trees should be planted down the center of the street with a roadway on each side. The facades of the houses are clear to the sunlight, easy to access, and the trees can develop in a uniform fashion."[44] Large avenues like the Avenue de la Marine in Tunis were modeled after similar throughways in Paris, such as the Avenue des Champs-Elysées.[45] Owing to the height of the street-facing buildings and a high flow of traffic, these thoroughfares were built with an island of trees in the middle of the street and an additional island of trees flanking each side of the avenue between alleyways and the sidewalk.

But it was not just lack of sunlight and air that made North African homes suspect. The interior courtyard, a signature feature of almost every residence, was considered "a den of vice into which kitchens and water closets emit their odors. Food is laid out in the courtyards where tenants shake out their carpets."[46] In many ways, it was not so much the lack of sunlight and air that disturbed the French as it was the confined closeness of constantly rubbing shoulders with one's neighbors while completing the most intimate tasks of cooking and bathing, which were often done in the courtyard. By the interwar years, privacy for carrying out bodily functions had become the norm in the West. Internal plumbing, hot water, and private bathroom facilities were de rigueur for middle class families. Those seeking admittance to bourgeois society needed to play by the rules of domesticity as arranged by the colonizer. French Jews were among the first to insist that Tunisian Jews would not, indeed could not, be accepted by polite bourgeois society if they insisted on living in overcrowded squalor. French hygienists stressed that dirty bodies and clothing should be dealt with in private; proper people do not air their dirty laundry (figuratively or literally) in public space. Historian J. P. Daughton has shown that French Catholic missionaries in the colonies have been incorrectly described as forces of a "distinctly 'modern,' bourgeois form of European hegemony."[47] Although this claim may hold true for Catholic missionaries, French Jewish activity in the colonies, especially as represented by the AIU, was unflinching in its appeal to modernity and steadfastly bourgeois in tone.

French bourgeois notions of domestic space required that each room serve a purpose corresponding to its name. For example, the bedroom housed the bed and was specifically designated as a space for sleep, quiet, and intimate sexual relations. Guests are received in the living room or salon, and eating is done in the dining room. By the interwar years, kitchens and bathrooms could be found in most French bourgeois homes. Even though regulations required "a well-lit and well-ventilated lavatory for every house, or for each apartment, that contains more than three rooms," most Tunisian Jews lived in one cramped room.[48] Families—husbands, wives, grandmothers, nephews, maiden aunts, widower uncles, and children of all ages—lived, slept, ate, and carried out intimate acts in the full view of other family members. No one had privacy, and bourgeois notions of modesty were unknown.[49] Nevertheless, French experts, like Charles Nicolle of the Institut Pasteur de Tunis, insisted on a unique link between modern sanitary reform and bourgeois domesticity, which initiated programs both on a grand public scale and in the private confines of the middle-class home.[50] Nicolle made the important connection between typhus and cleanliness when he noted that patients at the Sadiqi hospital in Tunis who were routinely stripped of their clothing and bathed failed to contract typhus at the same rates as others in the hospital, like laundry workers. The direct correlation between cleanliness and disease mitigation—the link between the flea and its host—was undeniable.[51]

Sewers, Water, Fresh Air, and Sunshine: Regenerated Communities

> In many cases, the poverty and laziness of the indigenes make their houses the receptacle of various fermentations. The colonist cannot live in good health unless these houses of infection are destroyed. Cleansing the indigenous quarter is one of the first tasks to undertake and it is even urgent to do it rapidly when these quarters are located in town. This cleansing will force the population density of the indigenous people to limit itself, overcrowding being more dangerous here than in France. We must build tree-lined avenues, with streets built to accommodate running water and sewer lines.[52]

French officials, fronted in the early years of the Third Republic by idealists, like Jules Ferry, and later by more money-wise politicians, like the Ministères des Colonies Henri Simon and Albert Sarraut, recognized the financial and logistical difficulties inherent in the implementation of their goals in regard to the *mission civilisatrice*, most notably in the realm of urban public health.[53] However, in Tunis and other "Arab" cities of the Maghrib, the goals of extending hygienic reforms to the colonial masses ran counter to desires to preserve the medina with all of its quaint eccentricities that attracted Western gawkers. In the mid-nineteenth century, Tunisia became a favorite destination for the European elite to winter and was also a peripheral stop on the Grand Tour. In 1895 Thomas Cook & Son commercialized travel to Tunisia when it included Tunisia as part of a package holiday to North Africa. In the late nineteenth century, tourism was emerging as an industry that could not only make money but also spread French prestige. The protectorate created the Office du Tourisme Tunisien to help the French get to know their empire and witness firsthand the stark contrasts between the indigenous way of life and French modernity.[54] One reason for the metropolitan government's recalcitrance toward funding hygiene and sanitation projects in Tunis was the fear that modern intervention in the Tunis medina would alter its historic nature. Where reorganization of the city of Tunis was concerned, French urban planners recognized that there was a tension between those who wanted to modernize and cleanse Tunis and those who wanted to preserve "historical" Tunis. The installation of sewers and water lines or the destruction of unsanitary structures could not, according to the Quai d'Orsay (French ministry of foreign affairs), interfere with the Oriental charms of the "Arab" quarter. Western travelers and settlers fetishized the Kasbah and medina as discrete locations of indigenous authenticity.[55] To the French, the Arab quarter represented a site of mystery, sensuality, and excitement; it was an unknown and unknowable world that epitomized the inscrutability of domestic life in the Maghrib.

French policymakers, especially in the Quai d'Orsay, embraced and encouraged the stereotype of Arab recalcitrance to innovation and hoary obscurantism and cynically juxtaposed them to the meme of Jewish cooperation and assimilation. In the view of the French administration, colonial communities that were politically stable and amenable to change, like the Jewish community of Tunis, were well suited to modernization projects and wholesale acculturation. However, Algeria had taught the French a valuable lesson about avoiding metropolitan overreach in regard to soliciting support from Maghribi Jewry. Although Muslims did not particularly want to be embraced by "French modernity," especially when that meant altering religious tenets, such as renouncing shari'a law in favor of French civil law, Muslims did not want Jewish interests promoted to the detriment of the Muslim population either, as they claimed had been the case after the Crémieux Decree's mass naturalization of Algerian Jews in 1870.[56] Similarly, French settlers jealously guarded their status as "Frenchmen" in the colonial hierarchy and were unwilling to surrender claims to this vaunted status to indigenous Jews. This jealousy prompted several outbreaks of violent anti-Semitism in Algeria that Tunisia (and later Morocco) sought to avoid.[57] Therefore, in Tunisia the protectorate regime avoided sweeping reforms to the civil status of the indigenous population.[58] The government weighed carefully the interests of colonial policies "favoring" Jews against the alleged detriment of such policies to both indigenous Muslims and French settlers.[59] The decision by French protectorate officials to strictly limit the number of Muslims naturalized as French citizens gave credence to those who viewed social and political discord through an ethno-religious lens.[60] Nevertheless, the preservation and "safeguarding" of Arab neighborhoods through a policy of benign neglect, for the most part, appeased both indigenous Muslims and French settler communities. Henceforward, the primary debate shifted to Jewish areas and the extent to which modernization could be pursued while maintaining the civil and social status quo preferable to Muslims and French settlers.

The Jewish quarter, or hara, was woven into the fabric of the Arab medina. The hara of the early twentieth century and interwar years was an area of extreme poverty that knew few ethnic or religious distinctions. Jews were no longer legally bound to dwell within its confines (it is debated whether or not they ever had been), and poor Muslims and Christians moved in to occupy the former dwellings of Jews who had moved up socioeconomically and left the quarter. However, in spite of its ethnic and religious diversity, the hara maintained its historical legacy in the minds of the *tunisois* as a distinctively Jewish space, and colonial officials, who ardently opposed blurred "racial" boundaries, willingly accepted this categorization. The hara was Jewish space; the remainder of the medina was "Arab."

Areas that were inscribed as rich in "Arab" history and tradition would be preserved; all else could be reorganized. In the colonial mind, Jews were not Arabs—at least, not in the culturally meaningful ways that Muslims were. Those Jews who did not reach a level of acculturation to be considered French (which was the majority) occupied a liminal space in the colonial world. Marginalized Jews, especially those in the hara, formed a separate identity group in the minds of their assimilated brethren, and indeed even in their own minds. Although they were not French, they certainly were not Arab.[61]

Even the poorest Jews in the hara fervently began to distinguish themselves from the "Arabs" in their midst. The ways in which marginalized Tunisian Jews perceived their own identities is laid bare in the following excerpts from the book *Jewish Memories*.[62] Tita S. lived among the poorest Jews in the hara, yet she and her family regarded themselves as members of an exclusive set. When asked how her mother dressed, Tita S. replies that her mother dressed in "a *sarwal* and a handkerchief like mine." For clarification, the interviewer asks if Tita's mother wore a veil, to which she adamantly replies, "No. We're not Arabs!" Similarly, when she recalls gatherings in the house's courtyard, Tita S. is asked if she sat on the ground while talking with her company. Tita S. insists, "Standing. We didn't sit down. Are we Arabs?" Throughout her interview, Tita S. refers to French speakers as "Monsieur" and "Madame," yet collectively refers to all Tunisian Muslims as "Arabs," never once naming one as an individual.[63] In her mind, the Arabs formed a collective, monolithic bloc that was antithetical to the recently articulated "modern" Jewish lifestyle so closely associated with France. Even though she and her family were reduced to the extreme penury of the hara, they nonetheless differentiated their behaviors from those of the Arabs and elevated the status of all things French.[64]

This brief excerpt also vividly demonstrates the complicated and shifting nature of identity politics in colonial Tunisia. Poor Jews, now freed from the humiliation of *dhimmi* status, envisaged themselves as not just religiously different from Muslim Tunisians but as socially different from Arabs. In fact, the term "Arab" to describe a Muslim Tunisian was a construct coined and disseminated during the colonial era. But just as the word "Arab" was used by Tunisian Jews to define what they were not, Tunisian nationalists increasingly used the word to describe what they were. "Arab" became a term increasingly linked to opposition of the French colonial domination of Tunisia. For Jews to be modern and French, it was essential that they reject the "Arab" side of their cultural identities in order to fully politically and socially align with the French. Importantly, working out the definitions of what it meant to be French and determining the behaviors and values that would constitute proper expressions of "Frenchness" often occurred *outside* the borders of continental France.[65]

At the same time, the French differentiation between Arabs and Jews increasingly attributed a cultural difference to what indigenous Tunisians had always considered a religious distinction. In many ways, cultural differences became a proxy for perceived racial and religious variances in the French Maghrib.[66] Colonial officials seized on and exaggerated these differentiations. According to the French paradigm, "old" Jewish space and traditions were not worthy of historical preservation; Jewish space was ripe for regeneration. After all, only "Arab" space was authentic to the Orient, and that is what merited preservation. The hara could—and would—be razed with impunity. As described movingly in Memmi's works, Jews occupied an inexorable no-man's-land in French colonial society.[67] Regardless of how Jews viewed themselves, the French and Muslim Tunisians agreed increasingly on one point: Tunisian Jews were neither wholly French nor Arab. "Jew" became an identifier stripped of its intrinsic cultural value, one that deserved no consideration regarding preservation of heritage.

During the great modernization and housing boom of the interwar years, the French administration made clear that it expected to recast Tunis as a segregated city while preserving the nature of the medina. To ensure social and domestic harmony, urban planners advocated the separation of races, faiths, and social classes into discrete residential pockets.[68] The oval-shaped medina represented the nucleus of Tunis and, aside from the Jewish hara, was seen as an untouchable zone of Arab authenticity.[69] As we have seen, protectorate officials hesitated to enact any hygienic measures that could alter its charms. In another dramatic example, although the city of Tunis decreed the mandatory use of trash cans, the indigenous quarter (the medina and Kasbah) was exempted from these regulations.[70] Trash cans were necessary in areas where colonists carried out their daily lives but not needed in areas where the French could "slum" in native authenticity.[71] Surrounding this nucleus of indigenous and untouched authenticity, protectorate officials envisaged an array of orbiting suburbs whose population would be determined by religion, "race," and class.[72]

Before exploring further how French officials executed their plans to redraw the map of Tunis, we must first consider the legal reforms that made urban and suburban reorganization possible. In the early nineteenth century, Tunisia had adopted many of the liberalizing Ottoman Tanzimat reforms; however, the strong Islamic tradition that governed land use and ownership in Tunisia remained intact. When the protectorate was established in 1881, property law in Tunisia was still administered by shari'a courts, which proved to be a major bone of contention to the French settler community. French settlers, daunted by the complex bundle of rights governing the possession and use of real property under shari'a law, sought to dispense with the system altogether. They argued that the land titling system in Tunisia was imprecise, incomplete, and often in conflict with other previously recorded documents.[73] Settlers, backed by the protectorate, argued that clear title to land, preferably in fee simple, was vital to prove ownership, quash competing claims, and dismiss legal uncertainty. According to Western-trained legal scholars, allowing tracts of property to be recorded by Islamic 'ulama who were untrained in the complexities of cartography and land platting stymied economic growth, led to uncertainty of ownership, and most important, was unfair to outsiders unacquainted with the intricacies of shari'a law.[74]

To guarantee Tunisia's ultimate success as a "modern" and productive state under the tutelage of French settlers, protectorate officials gave much attention to reforming and eliminating the complexities of shari'a-based property law and land tenure systems in Tunisia. Although the foundation of the Tunisian legal system in the precolonial era rested on a vast network of overlapping and even competing juridical sources, the crux of property law rested on the long-held belief of God as the ultimate landowner, as well as on an ethos of redistributive fairness.[75] In the view of colonial officials, the uncertainty of this shari'a-inspired legal paradigm was antithetical to rational land use and a market-based division of scarce land resources.[76] In short, the socioeconomic equity, sharing, and fundamental fairness that governed property rights and land use under shari'a law were a poor substitute for the legal certainty and clarity provided by Western legal systems.

To facilitate land acquisition by French settlers, French officials took a page from imperial Britain's playbook and adopted a Torrens system of land registration in 1885, which shifted all prior questions regarding possession of clear title in Tunisia from Judicial Services to the Directorate of the Interior.[77] Under the Torrens system, the central governing authority—in this case, the protectorate's Directorate of the Interior—recorded the ownership of land in a central registry, which established ipso facto absolute ownership rights to the real property in question. Moreover, in a Torrens system, any transfer or rerecording of ownership in the central registry sufficiently effectuates the conveyance of real property; there is no deed that changes hands. The Torrens system, although short on equity, is highly effective in its ability to dispossess indigenous landholders and extinguish prior legal claims to real property, especially in new settler communities.[78]

By vesting the power of recording land ownership in a newly created central government authority, the protectorate jettisoned the shari'a system *and* circumvented the requirement for settlers to prove clear title. This reform cleared the way for the gradual dissolution of *habous* lands and eliminated the necessity for French administrators and colonists to understand the complexities of Islamic property law.[79] Furthermore, all appeals regarding property rights would now be made in the first instance to the Court of Appeals (Cour d'Appel) in Algiers and ultimately to the French Supreme Court (Cour de Cassation) in Paris.

Now legally debarred from planning neighborhoods on "unused" or "empty" property, the protectorate launched construction on the first of the inner-ring suburbs, Franceville, just before the outbreak of World War I. This was followed after the war by the construction of Mutuelleville. These suburbs, flanking the southern and northern side of Parc du Belvédère respectively, were built to house French civil servants.[80] Just adjacent to Mutuelleville, to the west and north, were the Jewish planned-communities of Crémieuxville and Beau-Site. Protectorate authorities often worked hand in hand with assimilated Jews to create these middle-class enclaves. Beau-Site was created "thanks to a coordinated and insistent effort led by former instructors of the AIU."[81] These two communities, Crémieuxville and Beau-Site, were also reserved for civil servants, but of the Jewish faith. Middle-class French in Mutuelleville and Jews in neighboring Crémieuxville and Beau-Site shared the unifying characteristics of belonging to the same social class but were relegated to segregated enclaves as members of different faiths. Although Mutuelleville was adjacent to two Jewish communities, it was separated from Crémieuxville to the north by an open-air canal/sewer (*khandak*) and from Beau-Site to the west by a wide outer-belt-style avenue.

In a similar fashion, the protectorate also planned communities for "working-class" French settlers.[82] La Cagna was located on the far south side of town and respectively designated for French veterans and French postal and railway workers.[83] The working-class French neighborhoods were constructed well south of the city beyond the Cimetière El Jallaz (formerly Cimetière de Sidi Bel Hassen), the largest Muslim cemetery in Tunis, in an apparent effort to distance blue-collar French from the indigenous population.[84]

Although housing for Muslims always seemed to occur as an afterthought to protectorate officials, the government did build two enclaves for "Tunisian civil servants of the Muslim faith," Taoufik and El Omrane. The Taoufik project was quite small but appropriately located, nestled up against the western edge of the medina and Kasbah. Although the El Omrane quarter for Muslim white-collar workers enjoyed a privileged location on the south side of the Parc du Belvédère, it was separated kitty-corner from French-inhabited Franceville by two wide thoroughfares. Like the separate but equal Jewish and Christian communities north of the park, the Muslim and Christian communities south of the Parc du Belvédère existed side by side as economic equals but separated by the wall of faith (see map 3).

The division of the population according to religion and, more significant, social class is evident. Blue-collar workers resided south of the city's

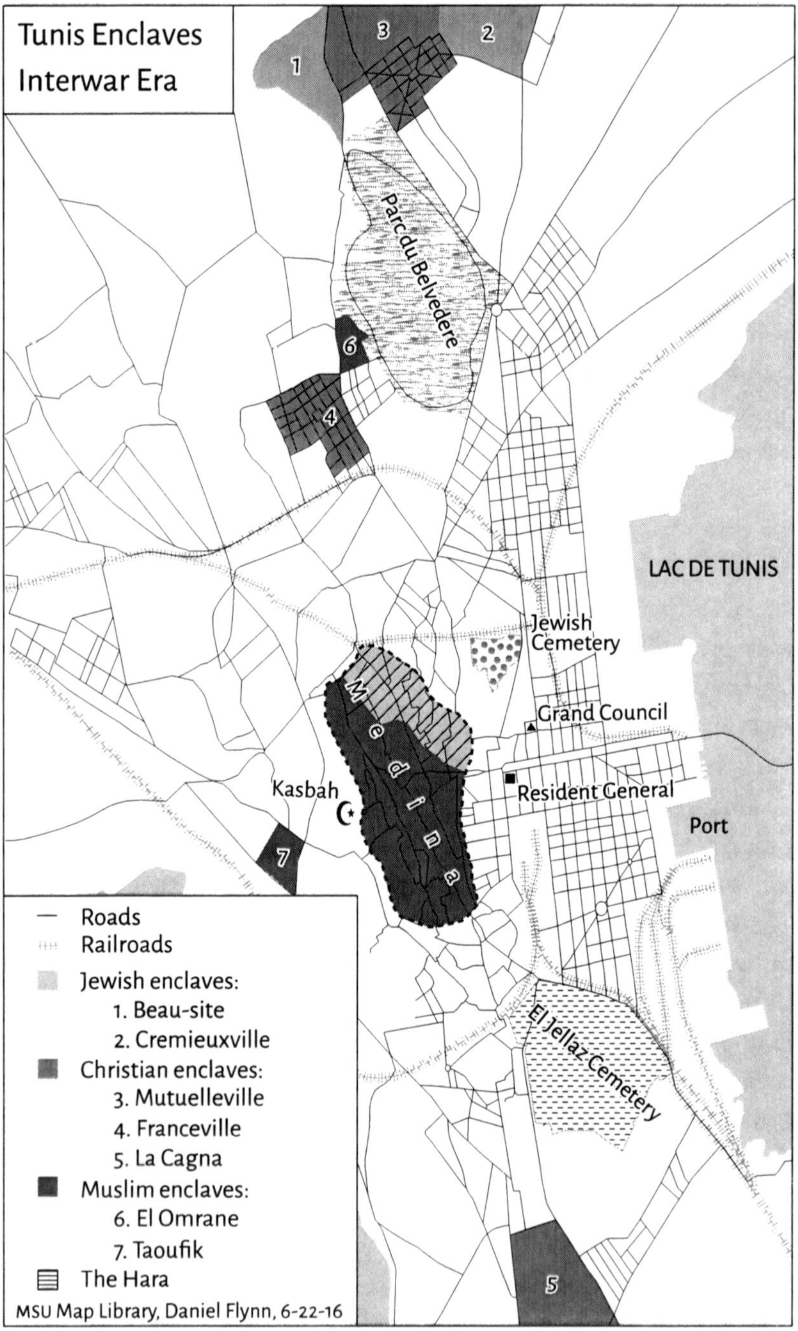

MAP 3. Tunis enclaves, interwar era. Created by Daniel Flynn.

nucleus, whereas the north side was reserved for "white collar" *functionnaires*. In each of the examples, Jews, Christians, and Muslims of the same class were "equal" enough to live in contiguous communities provided that they were "separated" by readily identifiable physical boundaries.

To demarcate further each enclave, the protectorate designated the streets with names that were intended to please (and identify) the intended inhabitants. For example, the streets in the French white-collar areas (Franceville and Mutuelleville) were given names such as Rue Descartes, Rue Baudelaire, Rue Clemenceau, and Rue de Cherbourg. In the French blue-collar neighborhoods south of the city, the streets were named for metropolitan steel districts (Rue de la Meurthe, Rue de la Sarre) and French military outposts (Rue du Cambodge). Similarly, streets in Jewish neighborhoods, such as Crémieuxville and Beau-Site, were named after the heroes (French, not indigenous) of the Jewish community, such as Zola and Abbé Grégoire, and for "Oriental" cities with large Sephardi populations, such as Smyrna and Rhodes. Streets in the Muslim enclaves were named (in transliterated French) after notable figures in Muslim history and literature, such as Rue al-Farabi and Rue Amine Arraihani.[85]

The amount of land that each ethno-religious group was allotted per resident was another characteristic of distinction between the neighborhoods. Looking at the number of hectares allotted per house in the interwar year plans for each area, Muslim areas were by far the most densely populated with only 0.088 hectares per housing unit. Jews and Christians fared the best: Jews with 0.132 hectares per housing unit and Christians with 0.160 hectares per house, nearly double the amount of space allotted to Muslims. Even when the prewar plans for Franceville are included in the statistics, Christians still got 0.129 hectares per housing unit, which was about the same amount of land apportioned to Jews and drastically more than that allocated to Muslims.[86]

In the fall of 1911, a municipal council plan to survey the al-Jellaz Muslim cemetery for possible redevelopment provoked protests and clashes with police that killed eleven people, seven of whom were police officers.[87] As a result of fervent opposition and to show respect to Muslim sentiments, the French abandoned any plans to alter the cemetery or "relocate" the dead. But it was not just dead *Muslims* who presented obstacles to the orderly blueprints of French urban planners—the land occupied by Jewish cemeteries also came under scrutiny.

Located on a parcel of land wedged between the Avenue de Londres and the Avenue Roustan—its northeast corner touching the area *tunisois* call *"le passage"*—the Jewish cemetery in central Tunis, the Ancien Cimetière, occupied an area of ever-increasing commercial and residential activity. Originally located on the outskirts of Tunis, the Ancien Cimetière (also called the Cimetière Bethe Ahaim Ier) housed the dead of both of Tunis's Jewish communities, the indigenous Twansa and the Livornese Grana. However, by the 1930s the Avenues de Londres and Roustan, which formed the peripheral boundaries of the Ancien Cimetière, had become the center of a thriving neighborhood. The Passage is a bustling commercial and residential sector sandwiched on a sliver of land east-northeast of the medina extending off the northern edge of the *ville nouvelle*. It is also the intersection of commuter rail lines that connect various sections of the city of Tunis.

As seen from a bird's eye, the footprint of the cemetery followed the rectilinear patterns of the new French-style residential streets popping up around it, except for one notable exception: *la hernie de l'avenue Roustan* (the Avenue Roustan hernia). Although the Avenue Roustan traced a straight line on its way to *le passage*, the cemetery itself bulged outward, blocking southbound lanes of traffic, which caused bottlenecks of cars, donkey carts, and pedestrians. The French administration decided that it must operate on the hernia to ensure the smooth and efficient flow between downtown Tunis, including the medina, and the salubrious, residential areas to the north. Although the specific objectives of sanitarians and urban planners were often at odds, there were moments when the goals of public health and traffic abatement aligned, and both interests could "share a conviction in the virtue of unimpeded circulation for the healthy urban body."[88] And as urban planners and hygienists described the irregularities of the urban structure of the hara in medical terminology, the Jewish cemetery inscribed the muscular weakness, or hernia, of Jews on the topography of Tunis itself. The hernia did not call for wholesale destruction like the hara but for a surgical procedure.

Although the French planned to act immediately, they wanted to frame the seizure of the property and suppression of the bulge as a legal act. That there was no clear title to the land in question hampered their efforts. In 1901 the Jewish charity agency le Comité de Secours et de Bienfaisance des Israélites represented by its president, Isaac d'Elie Nataf, sought permission from the municipality of Tunis to register title of the property occupied by the cemetery in the name of the charitable organization.[89] The municipality refused to register title to the organization, and the organization sued to establish its right to clear title. The court rejected the claim on two counts. First, the court was unable to establish clear prior title to the land in question. In other words, the court could not transfer title from an unknown party. Furthermore, representatives of the Twansa community had filed the instant case, and members of the Grana community claimed that as members of the Jewish community at large they should possess, at the very least, partial rights to the real property in question. Interjecting itself into the internecine strife between rival Jewish communities was not something for which the court had much enthusiasm. Hence, the court hedged its decision to refuse title to the charitable group by holding that as a charitable entity, it did not possess the personal jurisdiction requisite under Tunisian law to possess real property. The court recognized that several entities claimed title to the property and buildings on the site of the Ancien Cimetière. As the court had resolved the issue at hand—whether le Comité de Secours et de Bienfaisance des Israélites could register title to the property—any further questions as to the disposition of or clear title to the property were held in abeyance. In 1901 there were matters more pressing than who possessed clear title to a Jewish cemetery on the outskirts of Tunis.

As the neighborhoods surrounding the cemetery grew and the Passage became a thriving commercial area, the lingering question of who held title to the cemetery became increasingly important. In early 1930 the protectorate government decided that the hernia of the Avenue Roustan must be surgically removed from the map of Tunis and requested that the Jewish community acknowledge the city's right to remove the obstruction. The members of the Conseil de la Communauté Israélite, who had just gone through a bruising election campaign wherein one of the most contentious issues had centered on the fate of the cemetery, adamantly refused. In spite of this refusal, the French government claimed that for reasons of "passive defense" and the security of Tunis, the time for talk was finished, and the land was seized.

In a handwritten addendum, the *Directeur de l'Administration Générale et Communale* wrote that "the hernia must be strangled off" and that to "avoid a farce," the government intended to act "within the fortnight."[90] Once the government made its decision, it acted with alacrity. On March 28, 1939, over vociferous protests from the Jewish community, construction crews began the effort to remove the curved exterior wall of the cemetery and bring it more in line with the urban design of the French *ville nouvelle*.

Multiple examples in this chapter demonstrate how the French protectorate regime used public health codes and urban planning to remap life in Tunis, Balkanize communities, and regenerate Jews. In a city where Jews and Muslims, especially over the preceding two centuries, had lived cheek by jowl, the French instituted segregation, not only along "racial" and religious lines but also according to class. The razing of the historical Jewish quarter and the safeguards placed on "Arab" areas intensified these divisions. Jews, as shown by the destruction of the hara and the hernia, were forced to yield to modernity in a way that "Arabs" were not.

The French expressed and fetishized the exoticism of the Arab Orient in myriad ways: the art of Delacroix, Gérôme, and Ingres; Flaubert's *Salaambô*; the popular comic books *Les Aventures de Tintin*; Napoleon I's Egyptian campaign; Empress Eugénie's inauguration of the Suez Canal; and the popular travel narrative *Voyage en Orient* by Nerval, to name but a few. In the nineteenth and early twentieth centuries, the French public commoditized and consumed the Orient on a daily basis. The Orient satisfied the prurient desire of Western Europeans to gawk at and be titillated by the souks, the *hammams*, and the harems. But the outward manifestations of the traditional Oriental way of life centered on Muslims: the minarets, the call to prayer, the veiled women cloistered in courtyards impenetrable to Western eyes. Although Tunis was a Muslim-minority city during the interwar years, traditional Oriental space in Tunis continued to be closely associated with Islam.[91]

According to the view of the "Islamic city" popularized by the architectural historian Georges Marçais, urban areas in North Africa were not only indelibly linked to Islam; they also held traces of a lost chapter in the histories of Rome and Christendom.[92] In Marçais's Weltanschauung, ninth-century Arab architecture bears a striking resemblance to French Romanesque architecture, minarets hearken back to Roman watchtowers, and the aisles of the mosque that run parallel to the *qibla* wall (the prayer wall facing Mecca) draw their inspiration from the Christian basilica.[93] The view of the Islamic city as a historic relic and, moreover, a repository of early Christendom's artistic and architectural influence redoubled French efforts to preserve these "authentic" features of the medina. Of course, subsequent scholarship has shown that much of Marçais's assertions were based on a rather myopic Gallocentric view of history. Furthermore, like many other scholars of his period, he conflates Jewish expression as either "Arab" or considers it of little value. Much of this view that discounts Jewish urban life in the Maghrib, or that lumps it as part of "Arab" history, has been dispelled by recent work regarding Jewish life in the Islamic cities of North Africa.[94] For example, the dissolution of ancient relationship patterns of those living inside the Jewish quarter of Marrakesh, the *mellah*, and those on the exterior reveal the history of how Muslims, Jews, and French colonists negotiated space in Marrakesh as the colonial structure altered historical patterns of social, political, and economic behaviors.

Of course, the paradigm of the Islamic city as a space of authentic historicity relies heavily on the view of France as the defender and disseminator of modernity. But as an historical or indeed conceptual category, "French modernity" is a slippery term. "Modernity" is a multifaceted word that implies different meanings to different people. To some, it suggests the simplification or elimination of redundant, time-consuming tasks through industrialization, mechanization, and technological innovation. However, to others, the discourses of modernity—framed around an understanding of society's dialectical relationship to its environment—portend the dramatic alteration and rationalization of space, the transmogrification of the physical body, and the socio-moral transformation of backward, obsolete ways of thinking and being. As will become more clear in the following chapter, French officials—encouraged by French Jews and eagerly joined by elite Tunisian Jews—actively accepted and then pushed this latter, more invasive form of the modernization project on economically disadvantaged Tunisian Jews. French colonial officials and their allies hoped to achieve the comprehensive physical and moral regeneration and modernization of indigent Tunisian Jews—both through the corporeal transformation of Jewish bodies into French men and the total spatial reorganization and *embourgeoisement* of the hara into French space.

In the late nineteenth century, Jews and Muslims shared the neighborhoods of Tunis; however, the enforcement of colonial segregationist practices under the regenerationist guise of public health and urban reforms halted and reversed this trend between the First and Second World Wars. The mid-nineteenth-century scientific discoveries of bacteriology and the germ theory of disease, coupled with the rise of new disciplines like urban planning and sanitary science, reinvigorated and modified the allegory of regeneration from its origins in late eighteenth-century Enlightenment philosophy. Technocratic experts steeped in the scientific and medical intricacies of modern public health represented regeneration as a social and biological fact. Armed with this scientific authority, French officials thwarted what they perceived as the two greatest threats to their supremacy in Tunisia: inferior numbers and indigenous unity. As a direct result of policies to combat these threats, French urban reforms erased the continuities of multicultural Tunis and rehoused the population into discrete zones based on ethnic, religious, and class distinctions.

Sweeping public health reforms and strict urban planning promoted by both medical authorities and sanitarians justified French regeneration efforts that effectively neutralized both internal and external threats to French supremacy in Tunisia. By Balkanizing Jews and Muslims into economic, social, and religious enclaves, French authorities stymied the collaboration between Jews and Muslims in indigenous nationalist movements, and by destroying Jewish neighborhoods and recasting Jews as "regenerated" French citizens, for the first time in 1936, the French population finally surpassed that of the Italians. As the world hurled toward the cataclysm of World War II, the French, in their view, had finally gained the upper hand in Tunisia.

3 Regenerating Space, Part 2

Not All Ghettoes Are the Same

Just as I sat on the fence between two civilizations, so would I now find myself between two classes; and I realized that, in trying to sit on several chairs, one generally lands on the floor.

—ALBERT MEMMI, *The Colonizer and the Colonized*

As we saw in the prior chapter, the French regime selectively used the scientific and medical authority of public health and hygiene to redraw the map of Tunis—separating the city's neighborhoods along ethnic, religious, and class boundaries. By casting "Arab" areas as indigenous spaces of inherent value, much of the medina and Kasbah remained untouched by intrusive health and hygienic regulations, while areas of "no historic value," like the French *ville nouvelle* and neighboring La Goulette, were highly regulated and subjected to invasive intervention. In this chapter I will discuss the one area of Tunis to which I paid scant attention in the prior chapter: the hara. The Tunis hara presented a special problem for those who wished to redefine Tunis's Jews as a modern, regenerated community that welcomed the cultural influence of France. The hara was ancient and Jewish, terms that were antithetical to the new and more desirable definition of Tunis's Jews as modern and French. This chapter describes how French and Tunisian Jews, together with public health officials, charted a course that would ultimately destroy the Tunis hara yet maintain an uncomfortable status quo in the Jewish quarter in central Paris. This chapter demonstrates the misguided use of public health ordinances in the pursuit of the chimerical vision of the regenerated colonial Jew. Furthermore, it shows the ways in which public health measures can be selectively enforced or ignored, both in the Muslim areas of Tunis and the Jewish areas of Paris, depending on the overarching governmental motivations. Whether in the metropole or the colonies, decisions, even when ostensibly guided by the concerns of detached science and medicine, were made and resources were spent where they could further the state's political and economic interests—be that the furtherance of Jewish cooperation in Tunis or the primacy of landowners in Paris. To underscore this fact, the themes of this chapter are analyzed through a geographical comparative framework. Objective science prompts hygienic reforms, yet we know that French authorities acted with a heavier hand in Tunis than in Paris. The stark contrast between urban reform movements in Tunis and in Paris highlights the important role of politics, money, and cultural power in the implementation of hygienic reforms and the elasticity of the regenerationist message. Comparing the reforms in Paris and Tunis shows that hygienic reform depended less on scientific and medical imperatives than on effective lobbying and the expenditure of political capital. But it also shows that science and medicine, even when ignored as objective reality, are still useful *as rhetorical devices* in marshaling political action.

Following the crushing defeat and tumult of the Franco-Prussian War of 1870, France slowly reclaimed her position as a political, economic, and cultural power on the world stage. Under the latest French iteration of republican democracy, the Troisième République, Paris emerged as the center not only of the new French republic but of a rapidly growing, often unwieldy empire. The large swaths of dark blue that demarcated the territorial expansion of the French Empire spread like wildfire through the Asian and the African continents.

Viewed from the cartographical level, the division of the world appeared neat and organized, even somewhat Copernican—the metropole represented the bright sun around which the colonial possessions revolved and from which they received the light and warmth necessary for their sustenance and growth. Colonial possessions that lay closest to metropolitan France, like the Maghrib, received the greatest benefit from the warming rays of metropolitan sun but were also subject to its harshest glare.

Few questioned the conventional wisdom that knowledge and civilization, including scientific and medical erudition, shone outward; the colonial planets, to continue our metaphor, generating no light of their own, were capable of only pale reflections of the center. In short, the superiority of France and the benevolent and civilizing influence she would exercise on those within her orbit was "common sense." Although there were voices from all sides of the political spectrum that questioned the economic and strategic benefits of empire, few, if any, questioned the superiority of French scientific and medical advancement and its potential to civilize and ameliorate the lives of "native" peoples.

Much of this overweening conceit—the confidence that France could bring a more rational, salubrious, and civilized existence to its colonial possessions—was founded on a steadfast belief in the power and authority of science and medicine. The timesaving benefits of modern conveniences and the promise of medically efficacious therapies inspired (ostensibly) awe and gratitude among the colonized and established a modicum of safety and order for the colonizer. The unidirectional flow of useful scientific and medical knowledge, from metropole to colony, was not in doubt. Given the remarkable technological, scientific, and medical advances credited to French researchers, the idea of a dialectical flow of information and knowledge, an intellectual conversation between metropolitan and colonial experts as equals, was inconceivable.

In 1931 France celebrated the one hundredth anniversary of its invasion of Algeria by hosting the International Colonial Exposition in Paris. At this self-congratulatory public relations extravaganza designed to showcase the jewels of its far-flung empire, France impressed on her people the tireless efforts required to extend civilization to the darkest reaches of the globe. The Tunis Municipal Council, eager to make Tunis known to the French metropolitan audience, arranged a "presentation of maps, photographs, watercolors, sketches, dioramas, and film," all aimed at "highlighting Tunis' development and embellishment during the 50 years of the French Protectorate."[1] However, in spite of the elaborately staged and highly exoticized depictions of life in Tunis that titillated spectators, the two cities—Paris and Tunis—actually shared a dirty secret. Each housed an overcrowded and insalubrious Jewish quarter whose very existence vexed its residents, sanitary engineers, and municipal officials.

A few weeks before the beginning of these festivities in Paris, the French protectorate, acting through the Tunis Municipal Council, offered its solution to "cleanse" the hara (Jewish quarter) of the medina (old city) of Tunis. In terms of hygienic conditions, physical infrastructure, and spatial layout the hara was virtually indistinguishable from the rest of the medina as a whole. French government officials, with the active cooperation of French Jews, pressured the Tunis Municipal Council to provide a lasting answer to the insalubrious and disordered environment that characterized the hara.[2] The solution was as dramatic as it was simple. Between May 1933 and the beginning of World War II, the Tunis Municipal Council expropriated and demolished the vast majority of the hara—twelve hectares (approximately thirty acres) in the heart of the medina—resulting in the displacement of an estimated twelve thousand people. City authorities proposed the construction of fourteen hundred "luxury" and eleven hundred "semi-luxury" apartments on the newly cleared land. However, by 1939 only three buildings housing four hundred Jewish families had been completed on the vast construction site, and all efforts were abandoned with the advent of war.[3]

One important "gift" that the French introduced to the indigenous people in their colonies was French urban planning and design. Only in the very recent past have historians taken up the task of dismantling the paradigm of the "Islamic city" and considering urban life in the Maghrib beyond nineteenth- and early twentieth-century Orientalist notions.[4] As a result of this reassessment of urban space in the Maghrib, scholars have expressed a newfound interest in the Jewish quarters of Maghribi cities, spurred by a confluence of interests in both the lives of Jewish communities in the Maghrib and the Jewish role, as disseminators and receivers, in the "civilizing" aspects of French colonialism.[5] In addition to scholarship on

French colonial urban planning in the major cities of Morocco, Algeria, and French West Africa, especially works that focus on the civilizing and assimilating aspects of French colonialism, more work has been directed of late at the sociocultural role of Jewish urban space.[6] Most of the early research on Jewish urban life under the French protectorate in Tunisia concentrated on the compilation of statistics but lacked any penetrating historical data analysis.[7] More recently, works on the marginal populations of Tunis have begun to address the lacunae of social history about Jews and other historically forgotten groups.[8]

In this chapter I continue that process and investigate the political and social environments in Paris and Tunis at a time of heightened anxiety concerning each city's Jewish ghetto, paying special attention to the scientific and medical rationalizations for regeneration and "cleansing." Examining the Saint-Gervais ghetto in Paris (also referred to as *le Marais* or *le Pletzl*) and the hara ghetto in Tunis, two dramatically divergent strategies of municipal sanitary intervention emerge. In Paris, city officials' approach to cleansing Saint-Gervais was halting, haphazard, and ultimately occurred under tragic circumstances during World War II. In contrast, the Tunis Municipal Council, at the behest of French and Tunisian Jews, acted swiftly and compassionately (at least in their view) to expropriate and raze the hara and rehouse the displaced Jews. Whereas the primary concern of Paris's municipal officials was maintaining the socioeconomic status quo of landowners and their wealthy allies, their Tunisian counterparts were envisioning a bold, almost utopian, Jewish quarter modeled on an idealized concept of French modernity and bourgeois domesticity.

Many Jews in the metropole were going through the same growing pains on the path to regeneration as their coreligionists in the colonies. Although science and medicine offered universally applicable remedies to the disorder called degeneration — systematic organization, cleansing, behavior modification, consistency through reason, and infrastructural reform — these solutions were not evenly adopted. To demonstrate clearly the disparate application of remedies on similarly situated communities, impoverished Jews in Paris and in Tunis, we must closely examine the vicissitudes of Jewish politics in the metropole and the living conditions within the Paris ghetto. This comparative framework lays bare how aborted progressive policies in the metropole were actively and aggressively pursued in the colonies and explores the justifications for these dramatic differences in the implementation of municipal urban renewal policy, along with the various interests that attempted to influence the debate. Although the introduction of public health measures and modern infrastructure through urban renewal are improvements (as far as health and safety are concerned), they are also "violently discriminatory" and disproportionally affect the poor, who are disenfranchised from the power structure.[9]

The Paris Ghetto

As explained in the introductory chapter, the condition of Jews in early twentieth-century France was extremely complex. Enlightenment era writings of the Abbé Grégoire, together with revolutionary and Napoleonic era reforms, had introduced France to the concept of Jews as fellow, equal citizens of the French nation. (Although as the Dreyfus Affair, Vichy collaboration, and right-wing extremism demonstrate, the concept that Jews are incapable of being loyal Frenchmen lingered [lingers] far beyond French "Enlightenment" and postrevolutionary reforms.) Many elite Jews found their voice in the Alliance Israélite Universelle (AIU)—an organization established in 1860 by a group of highly influential, wealthy French Jews. The goal of the alliance was to spread the message of the French Enlightenment to the "unenlightened" and to modernize, or "regenerate," the Jews of the Mediterranean basin. The impetus for this movement not only predates the Scramble for Africa but also traces its philosophical and political roots to eighteenth- and early nineteenth-century France.[10] Many members of the AIU successfully joined the ranks of the Parisian bourgeois elite, but in the view of French Christians, Jews and the ethnic enclaves that they inhabited remained suspect—a world apart. Stung by the suspicion and hatred of their fellow Frenchmen, elite French Jews preached to their brethren that they would only gain acceptance to French society through the "modernization" of their religious practices and Gallicization of their customs.[11] During the nineteenth century, elite French Jews increasingly distinguished semantically between the descriptors *Israélite* and *juif*. To many, the term "*juif*" was too closely associated with the negative terms "*juif errant*" (wandering Jew) or "*juif honteux*" (shameful Jew), and a new adjective that referred to Jews was needed. French Jews who successfully completed the societal and semantic journey from *juif* to *Israélite* achieved moderate gains in public and political acceptance, especially in Paris and Bordeaux. But in spite of the gains touted by Parisian Jews, including the founders of the AIU, the medieval legacy of suspicion and contempt remained an important facet of Christian-Jewish relations in France well into the twentieth century.

The postrevolutionary emancipation of Jews together with Napoleonic reforms had two important effects on French Jews, especially those in the upper classes. First, emancipation and liberal reforms heartened Jews to believe that they could now become part of the French nation. Second, these same reforms reified the idea among many Jews and Christians alike that Jews were irredeemable save through the glory of France. As elite Jews in France internalized the mythology of salvation and acceptance through unwavering allegiance to all things French, they proselytized the good news to their coreligionists and embarked on a mission to civilize backward French Jews.[12] In short, French Christians succeeded both in branding the Jewish community as retrograde and in demarcating Jewish space as a fertile point of insertion for French culture and assimilation.

Between the Franco-Prussian War (1870–71) and the reannexation of Alsace and Lorraine following World War I (1918), the demographics of the Parisian Jewish community underwent a sweeping change.[13] Jewish refugees from Central Europe, Poland (Russia), and Romania flooded into the Saint-Gervais district of central Paris—within steps of the Hôtel de Ville. The customs and behaviors of these new foreign arrivals alarmed Parisians, including many Parisian Jews, who for the most part had been absorbed into the economic and societal fabric of the capital. Parisians complained that newly arrived Jews espoused an ethnic solidarity that promoted disloyalty to country. A member of the Paris Municipal Council stated on record that he was opposed to the sort of "brotherhood" so characteristic of eastern Jews and that their presence only provoked divisions among the French people.[14] But potentially more infectious than their radical political views were the filth, disease, and strangeness that Parisians claimed accompanied these eastern Jews.

Medical authorities stressed a direct link between domestic hygiene and the future strength of the nation.[15] The ways in which refugees flouted the conventional rules of domestic conduct dismayed Parisians who had collectively agreed on a set of normative behaviors that these "others" seemed determined to violate. Their poverty and ignorance made them seemingly incapable of conforming to predetermined standards of hygienic and bourgeois "family values." Even more alarming than this breach of normative French bourgeois *moeurs*, these foreigners contributed, as officials complained, to France's most vulnerable weakness: demographic decline. Paris city councilmen noted that the Jews in the Saint-Gervais district represented an immediate danger to the hygiene and security of students at the nearby Charlemagne School for Young Ladies.[16] Another councilman complained that the offspring of these foreign-born Jews in Saint-Gervais were overwhelming milk dispensaries in neighboring arrondissements.[17] The French government, already frightened by low birthrates among *les Français de souche* (families of French stock), recognized that it must take action to preserve the health and welfare of France. Municipal councilors opined that the French government must force these "foreigners" to respect the hygienic laws and regulations of France. But the state, in the paralytic fashion typical of the Third Republic, pushed all responsibility back to municipal officials.[18]

With complaints rising and the ball lodged firmly in their court, the Paris Municipal Council was forced to confront the issue. One option that urban sanitation experts proposed—the total demolition of the lower Saint-Gervais quarter and re-housing of its overcrowded inhabitants outside Paris—appealed to many as a quick solution to the problem and, moreover, one with the added benefit of ridding Paris of the foreign Jewish danger. Local newspapers carried accounts advocating this "public health" approach: "We are talking about sordid foreigners, of undetermined nationalities whose excess of number create a danger for the health of the neighbors. What filthy promiscuity! We must cleanse these buildings, and send these masses, who are seeking direction, into camps in the vast suburbs."[19]

Indeed, in the first few decades of the twentieth century, reform-minded hygienists in Paris argued that the filthy, overcrowded areas of the city should be razed. They asserted that the removal of certain pre-identified "*ilôts insalubres*," or "pockets of pestilence," and a priori, of the filthy people who resided in them, would greatly benefit the overall health of the inhabitants of the entire city. Although most Parisians agreed in principle that ridding the capital of its pockets of pestilence was desirable, a potent force stood in the way of such dramatic intervention. Landowners and landlords represented a powerful lobby of wealthy individuals adamantly opposed to any interference by the government with their rights as property holders.

Property rights advocates adeptly reframed the public health debate in xenophobic terms: Why should "native Parisian" landlords have their properties destroyed because of the "filthy foreigners" who overcrowded them? Powerful Parisian landowners asserted that it was not their buildings that were toxic; it was the people who occupied them. They maintained that the solution to the problem was the wholesale removal of the unsavory tenants, not the destruction of the unhygienic structures. Although they realized that the removal of these tenants would be difficult, it was better than the alternative—demolition: "It would be quicker and more efficient if [Jewish workers] were not grouped in the same areas as their brethren. . . . A pick will be needed to force them to leave—this brutal solution would be an excellent alternative for them and a good in and of itself—for no one would support the demolition of nine-tenths of the neighborhood."[20]

In spite of this focus on the overcrowded inhabitants as the problem, hygienist presented counterevidence that overcrowding was actually far worse in non-Jewish quarters of Paris. In fact, even the people of Brittany, according to hygienic statistics, lived in worse squalor and teeming proximity than Paris's "foreign Jews."[21] The evidence, according to hygienic science, pointed to the buildings themselves—the lack of facilities and running water, crumbling infrastructure—as the true danger to public health and not the inhabitants per se. Yet the members of the Paris Municipal Council—many of whom owned buildings in the area in question—sided with the laissez-faire arguments of the property rights advocates over the view of the urban sanitation experts. A general lack of will, coupled with the refusal of landholding interests to cooperate with intrusive regulation, led the municipal council to water down its hygienic reform efforts. It acknowledged that razing insalubrious quarters was not a viable option after all; from now on, hygienists and sanitation experts should pinpoint discrete offending targets that would be "lanced like boils."[22] Cutting-edge science backed this "surgical" approach to slum clearance. While the prefect of the Seine, Georges-Eugène Haussmann, had relied on the miasmatic theory of disease etiology to justify sweeping infrastructural reforms and slum clearance in the mid-nineteenth century, by the turn of the twentieth century, medical science, now defined as bacteriology and the belief in disease caused by specific agents, required precise interventions to rid identifiable zones or even single buildings of noxious microbes.

Regardless of the debate between reform-minded hygienists and headstrong property owners, the extreme limitation of French expropriation laws would have greatly hindered the government from taking any potentially progressive or active reforms, such as forced condemnation and demolition of unhygienic properties. Expropriation in France was governed by the *loi de 1841*, which laid out the parameters of "expropriation for cause of public utility." As its title makes clear, this law anticipated the opening of new roadways or the execution of work for "public utility" only; it made no mention of the need to eliminate "households of infection" or the condemnation of property for public health concerns. Since the primary objective of the law was to *protect* private property, all expropriations required the unlikely approval of a jury of landowners.

In the wake of the staggering loss of life caused by World War I and the 1918 influenza epidemic, concern for public health and hygiene, if only to maintain France's population vis-à-vis its enemies, reached an apex. Hygienic reformers and sanitation experts urged the administration to revisit the *loi de 1841*. These progressive reformers argued that slumlords, who invest little or no money in their properties, ought not to earn, as a result, more money per square meter than a responsible landowner.

> In our society, it is a given that it pays to provide a service. But is it a service to offer the public rooms infected with tuberculosis and other diseases, aggravated by parasites that infest these places. Assuredly not. In all of these cases, the landlord has long since taken his compensation for any rendered services, and if he has only recently come into possession of such a building, he is a speculator and does not deserve any compensation for having believed that we would continue to tolerate this deplorable practice. The essence of the law, notably the guiding principles of commercial enterprise, agree that in the name of Justice and Morality the State can deprive land owners not of the right to own land, but of the abuse of that right, which is tantamount to a homicidal act. Hence, all dwellings that are "notoriously unclean" ought to be closed.[23]

Reacting to this groundswell of concern, French officials revised the *loi de 1841* to address the thorny issue of "*ilôts insalubres*." Sanitary officials hailed the resultant *loi de 1919* as a boon to public health—the new law anticipated the expropriation of properties deemed "manifestly dangerous to public health." Municipal officials would now ostensibly be able to clear slums in a wholesale fashion. But hygiene reformers quickly realized that the powerful lobby of property owners had duped them. Although the new law allowed for expropriation of property for reasons of danger to public health, it failed to replace the decision-making power of a "jury of landowners" with a more disinterested body.[24] In essence, property owners could band together to block any expropriation regardless of the proximity of the danger to public health presented by the offending property. In the final analysis, the long-awaited and much-lauded reformation of the expropriation law had little material effect on the Parisian ghetto or its unsanitary dwellings. Jewish neighborhoods in Paris, like Saint-Gervais, which had been almost entirely ignored by Haussmann's reforms in the mid-nineteenth century, were now pushed aside as a favor to wealthy landowners loath to deal with expensive material hygienic reforms.[25] The bottom line was that metropolitan Jews who enjoyed any influence or power preferred to spend their political capital abroad in the Jewish communities of the "Orient." The insular Parisian quarters occupied by downtrodden Jews were just not that politically important to French lawmakers and powerbrokers, whether Jewish or Christian. Even where public health and hygiene necessitated intervention, the concern, as a political imperative, was never formidable enough to provoke the requisite governmental response.

The French government ultimately "solved" the sanitary issues of the Saint-Gervais quarter, not out of a genuine concern for the health and welfare of its citizenry, but rather as the implementation of institutionalized and legalized anti-Semitic policies. Much of Saint-Gervais, so-called *ilôt insalubre no. 16*, was expropriated in 1941 and 1942 by the city's Office of Public Hygiene, which justified its intervention by reference to Vichy economic Aryanization laws.[26] In short, the Vichy regime replaced a hygienic crisis with a humanitarian one. French officials finally "cleansed" the overcrowded, filthy, substandard housing, not through progressive government intervention, but by forcibly depopulating the Saint-Gervais quarter, rebuilding it for Aryans, and "rehousing" the Jews in camps.[27] Even before Vichy, however, the health and welfare of the citizens of the Saint-Gervais quarter had never been the overriding concern of municipal officials; all debates over what to do in Saint-Gervais had centered on either the maintenance of property rights or expedient concerns over the lagging French birthrate. When a decision was finally made in regard to Saint-Gervais, the Vichy regime determined that it was the inhabitants who were the public health menace, not the crumbling infrastructure.

The Tunis Ghetto

The status of Jews in the French colonies was highly dependent on both the local customs and, in particular, how deeply the French intervened in preexisting social and political hierarchies. "Justice in Tunisia traditionally rested upon the fundamental principle that religious affiliation determined personal status under the law."[28] In early nineteenth-century Tunisia, Muslim rulers still classified Jews as *ahl al-dhimma*, or "protected people," and as such, the beys of Tunisia agreed to "protect" Jews (native Christians, also classified as "protected," had disappeared from the Maghrib in the Middle Ages) within their realm—for a price. Jews were subject to a yearly capitation tax, the *jizya*; forbidden to wear clothing reserved for Muslims, such as the red *chéchia* hat, white turbans, and colored shoes; and confined to the abject squalor of the hara—it is possible that they were required to do so until the 1870s.[29] One way that Jews could obtain a relatively secure legal status was under the protection of a European power. Many Jews involved in trans-Mediterranean trade obtained European "patents of protection."[30] However, I do not want to oversimplify the legal status of Jews in Tunisia. Even Jews who possessed a "patent of protection" did not hold the same rights and immunities as similarly situated Europeans; however, it was not unknown for both "protected" and "unprotected" Jews to get justice in Muslim courts. Nevertheless, in the main, Jews desired to avoid shari'a courts for what they viewed as a fairer alternative (a rabbinical court for intra-Jewish affairs, a European court, or during the protectorate, a "mixed" court). Jews who were protégés of a foreign power often had their cases deliberated concurrently in multiple jurisdictions or sought intervention by consular authorities.[31] By and large, it was the wealthiest Jews from commercial dynasties who could avail themselves of this option to escape the beylical legal system. To the vast majority of Jews in Tunisia, patents of protection remained unknown commodities.

Although the establishment of the protectorate regime (1881) ended the most shameful and egregious abuses against Jews and reduced the bey to a puppet of the French government, the arrival of the French administration offered the Jewish community in Tunisia a new and often illusory opportunity for "protection" through French naturalization. Although this vaunted status had been granted to Algerian Jews en masse by the 1870 Crémieux Decree, the French protectorate argued vehemently against the applicability of such a law in Tunisia.

> It is useless to insist upon the numerous inconveniences, even dangers that would arise by the adoption of a similar measure [i.e., a Crémieux Decree in Tunisia]. Not right now, while Algeria suffers from the advantages political parties were able to glean from the *décret Crémieux*, could we consider creating a similar privilege, however minimal it may be, for Jews in Tunisia in regard to the indigenous Muslims. All reform that would lead Jews in

> Tunisia down the path to assimilation with the French would create even more anti-Semitism in Tunisia as we have here [in Tunisia] 60,000 Jews and scarcely 16,000 French. . . . If ever assimilation, even partial, were allowed, the tiny French kernel would be completely drowned in the Jewish element.[32]

As the French solidified their hold on the administrative and legal apparatus, more and more indigenous Jews and Muslims expressed interest in accessing the benefits of French citizenship. In 1905 Mordechai Smaja published a brochure titled *L'Extension de la juridiction et de la nationalité française en Tunisie*, which he vigorously defended in his newspaper *La Justice*.[33] In spite of the support of the Frenchified segments of the Jewish population, the protectorate, as well as many conservative Jews, remained opposed to broad extension of French citizenship to Tunisian Jews. Many in the French government, particularly the anticolonial *revanchistes*, considered the Algerian Crémieux Decree of 1870 to have been a public relations and political disaster.[34] The French government argued that the naturalization of Jews created tensions between Jews and Muslims, between settlers and Jews, and also between conservative, religious Jews and French-acculturated, secular Jews. French officials also feared that the consolidation of the Tunisian Jewish community as French nationals under a sole consistory (*consistoire*) would lead to increased Italian influence if Grana money and influence swamped Twansa voices.[35] Jewish communities within France and her departments, such as Algeria, were divided into a network of consistories. Each consistory was under the aegis of the Central Consistory in Paris. As Tunisia was not divided into French departments but remained a protectorate, it had no consistories, which left Jewish communities in the hands of local leaders and rabbis who were not answerable to Paris. There exists no record of any Jew being naturalized as a French citizen between 1891 and 1910.[36]

Muslims countered that in lieu of granting citizenship to a select few, the entire judicial system ought to be reformed so that all Tunisians regardless of ethnicity or religion would be citizens of one state.[37] The Muslim position of course raises the question, citizens of what state:

France or Tunisia? In these claims for equal citizenship and treatment under the law lie the roots of the establishment of the Destour Party—a party that initially attracted some members of the Jewish intelligentsia.[38] The Destour Party, which sprang from the Young Tunisians, formed in 1920 and called for a restoration of the suspended 1861 Tunisian Constitution. At first many Destourians felt that the protectorate could be maintained so long as indigenous rights were expanded. There were some intellectual Jews who were attracted to this message. However, as the protectorate denied freedom of speech and assembly and eroded the jurisdictional purview of shari'a tribunals throughout the early 1930s, most Destourians eventually called for full Tunisian independence with a more Islamic bent. The turn from a secular rights-based party to a more Islamic-oriented party disenchanted Jewish adherents who abandoned the movement.

But the 1910 census of Tunisia conducted by the French protectorate showed a fact more alarming to the French regime than the incipient nationalist movements: in Tunisia the 105,000 Italian nationals grossly outnumbered the newly arrived 35,000 French settlers. As a result, on October 3, 1910, the president of France, Armand Fallières, issued a decree that extended French citizenship to Tunisian nationals who were fluent in the French language and fulfilled at least one of the following criteria: voluntary enlistment in the French military, academic distinction at a *grande école*, marriage to a French woman with resulting issue, more than ten years of "important service" to French interests in Tunisia, or "exceptional service" to France.[39] The selective and subjective nature of the new decree pleased few and made little sense. For example, one of the tenets of French citizenship was submission to the jurisdiction of French civil courts in all matters, including family law. Muslims considered the repudiation of shari'a jurisdiction as apostasy and maintained that Muslims who accepted French civil jurisdiction could no longer be buried in Muslim cemeteries. In spite of fatwas issued by both the Maliki and Hanafi muftis—under direct orders by Resident General Manceron—that ordered the religious burial of French Muslims in Muslim cemeteries, Muslims remained united against the regulation.[40] Jews also had little success in negotiating French citizenship from the new edict. Between the presidential decree of late 1910 and the Morinaud Law of 1923, only 299 Jews became naturalized French citizens.[41]

By the early 1920s the fear of the *péril italien* reached a fever pitch. Tunis had a significant community of Jews, called Grana, who had emigrated from Leghorn (Livorno, Italy) in the seventeenth century. These Jews spoke Italian, maintained their own rites, and were protégés, or even citizens, of Italy. With Mussolini's rise to power in 1922, the Italian conquest of Libya, and increased public proclamations by Italian statesmen that Tunisia was or ought to be part of Italy, the Quai d'Orsay issued further legislation in 1921, culminating with the Morinaud Law in 1923, which dismantled all Italian consular courts in Tunisia.[42] Italian protégé status or citizenship could no longer shield Grana Jews from the jurisdiction of the indigenous courts. Any Grana Jews who had not already been provoked by the Italian regime's increasing anti-Semitic rhetoric to surrender their claims to Italian protection or citizenship by their own volition were stripped of such rights by the protectorate in 1923. The calculated political move to beef up the number of Frenchmen in Tunisia through increased naturalization of hitherto "unwanted" Jews and Jews stripped of Italian patronage proved a successful method to shore up French power.

In addition to stripping Italian Jews of their Italian protégé status or citizenship, the Morinaud Law eased the prerequisites for French naturalization; however, the law still excluded the overwhelming majority of Tunisians. In reality, passage of the Morinaud Law was nothing more than a desperate attempt by France to win the demographic game in Tunisia vis-à-vis the Italians by granting French citizenship to select, wealthy *évolués*—mostly Jews. In the vernacular of French colonists and colonial officials, *évolués* had, through exposure to French language and education, "evolved" to a status higher than their "native" brethren. These "evolved" individuals, who embraced French cultural values and social norms, became the cornerstone of France's colonial policy of assimilation and were granted French citizenship on a case-by-case basis.[43]

Between 1924 and 1929, 4,873 Tunisian Jews, including Grana Jews who had been either Italian protégés or nationals, became naturalized

French citizens, and another 1,587 Tunisian Jews joined the French nation between 1930 and 1933. In part because of the French regime's volte-face on Jewish naturalization, in the Tunisian census of 1931 French citizens in Tunisia finally outnumbered Italians by 91,437 to 91,178.[44] Apparently, the French protectorate and the Quai d'Orsay calculated that Tunisia was better off "drowning" in a sea of "naturalized Jews" than being overrun by Italian fascists.

On the subject of Jewish naturalization, the protectorate was forced to walk a very fine line. On the one hand, the protectorate desired desperately to boost the number of French citizens in Tunisia, especially from among the Jewish population, both to create a bulwark against Italian claims on Tunisia, including those of the Grana Jews, and to splinter the "native" population by cleaving the Jews away from the Muslims. In fact, historian Yahya El Ghoul maintains that Resident General Lucien Saint in early 1921 viewed "the crisis of French population, the Italian problem, and the native problem" as interconnected and argued that by boosting the "French" population Tunisia would be easier to govern.[45] On the other hand, the protectorate and the Quai d'Orsay were also adamantly opposed to repeating the "Algerian mistake" of wholesale Jewish naturalization as instituted by the Crémieux Decree. For the French, the goal was to find a halfway point in the numbers of Tunisian Jews being naturalized as French, a number somewhere between the uncomfortable exclusion of Tunisian Muslims and the mass naturalization of Jews in Algeria.[46]

Although the loosened restrictions enabled the naturalization of 6,400 Jews between 1924 and 1933, the struggle to gain access to French citizenship or even just to secure basic legal and political recognition was too long and, in many respects, degrading for many Tunisians to stomach. Tunisians of all stripes were learning to express their political points of view through alternative outlets. Muslims and even some Jews turned to the growing Destour movement. Some Jews found their political voice in the expanding Zionist movement.[47] The number of naturalizations of Tunisian Jews plummeted to only 207 between 1934 and 1939. During the long wait for recognition, the seeds of alternative political discourse for indigenous Tunisians had been sown.

The statistical data revealing the sudden decrease in Jews seeking French naturalization after 1933 is also based on changing political events in Tunisia and France. Tunis in the early 1930s was experiencing a demographic explosion. As the deepening worldwide depression now affecting Tunisia drove small farmers off their land, impoverished displaced people flocked to Tunis. By the mid-1930s upward of 30,000 people in Tunis and 100,000 people nationwide were unemployed.[48] The regime's decision to subsidize settler's grapevines and fruit groves but not olive groves, which were largely in the hands of Tunisian small farmers, provoked a heated challenge to French authority. In 1933 elite Tunisians in the Grand Council joined with Destour forces led by Habib Bourguiba and called for noncooperation with the protectorate regime. With the backing of not only the Muslim intellectual elite but also small farmers, Bourguiba founded the Neo-Destour Party, effectively changing the tenor of Destourian class-based politics into Neo-Destourian identity-based politics with Tunisianness as the central rallying cry.[49] In these early days of Neo-Destourian politics, some influential Tunisian Jews, such as Élie Cohen-Hadria, were attracted to a party based on Tunisian national pride.[50] However, after a brief honeymoon period, ideas surrounding the emerging idea of Tunisian citizenship became more and more conflated with Islam and disenfranchised Jewish voices. In essence, most Jews were now excluded from both French citizenship and the "new" Tunisian identity based on Islam. Moreover, the fevered pitch of political rhetoric from Nazi Germany, Fascist Italy, and anti-Semites in France cooled the Jewish appetite for French citizenship, and the image of France as the standard-bearer for civilization and modernity suffered. In short, beginning in the late nineteenth century and culminating in the mid- to late 1930s, many disparate voices competed for the attention and loyalty of Tunisian Jews. However, the Jewish population of Tunisia was by no means monolithic, and the parties and groups through which they expressed their views were highly divergent, yet oddly many times overlapping. Where some Jews had flirted with the Destour Party and Zionism, others found political expression in communism and trade unionist activities.[51]

Whether Jew or Muslim, Zionist or Destourian, all groups shared a common home in the Tunis medina. Viewed from above, the medina of

Tunis occupies an oval-shaped parcel of land situated on the side of a gently sloping hill. On the western side, at the highest elevation, sits the Kasbah, the center of the indigenous government. The principal street bisecting the medina, rue de la Kasbah, slopes downward from the Kasbah to the Bab al-Bḥar (Door of the Sea, renamed Porte de France by French colonists). According to legend, at the close of the tenth century, Sidi Mahrez Ben Khalaf stood in the tower of the mosque now bearing his name in the northern section of the medina, surveying the growing city of Tunis. To parcel land fairly to Tunis's Jews, Sidi Mahrez repeatedly threw his staff from the top of the minaret; all areas within the holy man's throwing distance from the mosque's minaret would be set aside for Jews. His staff landed within the areas constituting the northeastern parts of the medina. This triangle shaped wedge of land, roughly bordered on the south by the rue de la Kasbah, the west by the rues Achour and Ettoumi, and to the north and east by the rue Bab Souika became the Jewish quarter: the hara.

Legend aside, historians know little about the establishment of the hara as a distinct Jewish quarter and debate whether Muslim rulers in Tunisia compelled Jews to live within a prescribed zone. It seems that the parameters of the Tunis hara were never as rigid as the boundaries of the Jewish quarters in Morocco, which were legally demarcated during the nineteenth century.[52] In fact, Jews in Tunis rented additional plots of land and buildings contiguous to the Jewish quarter in order to expand its size, and there exists no record of a wall or fence to contain the hara. Although it is unknown if Jews in Tunis were legally required to live within the hara, they likely did so of their own volition to benefit from the sense of community and limited self-governance promoted by their assemblage.[53]

Structurally, the hara was much like the rest of the medina: a multitude of low, whitewashed edifices built around sinuous paths, often blind alleys, many not wide or tall enough for a donkey cart to pass. But unlike the rest of the medina, the hara had long been considered a den of infection—more cramped, dirtier, and more suspect than the medina as a whole. This characterization was likely the result of latent anti-Jewish sentiment because no evidence exists that the hara was any more pestiferous than the rest of Tunis. Nevertheless, many Muslims claimed that Jews were responsible for bringing infection to the capital and propagating disease with their slovenly ways. During the colonial era, the reputation of the hara as a den of infection continued in spite of counterevidence. During the twenty years from 1909 to 1929, the rate of mortality per 1,000 citizens in Tunis was 23.57 among Jews (most of whom lived in the hara), but 36.42 among Tunis's Muslims (most of whom lived in the remainder of the medina).[54] A closer examination of morbidity and mortality statistics reveals that during the interwar era, death caused by infectious disease in Tunis was consistently higher among Muslims than Jews. In 1923 infectious disease accounted for 44.6 percent of deaths among Tunisian Muslims as opposed to 40.6 percent of Jews. The statistics for death from infectious disease in Tunis for the subsequent years are similar: 1924, 44.8 percent of Muslims and 44.7 percent of Jews; 1926, 44.4 percent of Muslims and 44.3 percent of Jews; 1927, 44.1 percent of Muslims and 41.3 percent of Jews; 1928, 42.3 percent of Muslims and 35.5 percent of Jews; and 1929, 45.8 percent of Muslims and 34.8 percent of Jews.[55] As these statistics show, by the post–World War I era, the allegation that Jews harbored infectious disease or were more susceptible to such diseases is not borne out by the numbers.

Nevertheless, French colonial officials, encouraged and led by elite French Jews in Paris (primarily members of the AIU), argued for drastic sanitary intervention in the hara. Although the latest theories of disease etiology had shifted to a "new public health," which relied on bacteriological precision and the specific targeting of infected individuals, colonial officials enthusiastically breathed new life into the miasmatic theory when it came to justifying massive infrastructural interventions.[56] Although new medical theories justified halting the wholesale destruction of neighborhoods in Paris, this was not the case in Tunis. More than willing to make the most of the hara's reputation as a hotbed of filth and disease, elite French Jews from Paris joined affluent Tunisian Jews and AIU teachers in calling for dramatic intervention.[57] Colonial officials lamented that it was far too difficult, if not impossible, to change the population's behavior and conduct more targeted cleansing operations. A better alternative to behavioral modification was expropriation and destruction of the hara in one fell swoop, even though it would be "very onerous to the population."[58]

Elite Jews in Paris, keenly interested in their Oriental coreligionists, joined forces with assimilated Tunisian Jews, who were represented on the Tunis Municipal Council, and agreed with this assessment. According to the Tunis Municipal Council, the hara ought to "be condemned to make place for a new European quarter, crossed by 35 meter wide thoroughfares from Porte de France to the Bab Bou Saadoun."[59] However, in the mind of the council, this "European quarter" would be occupied by Jews—rehabilitated and "regenerated" Jews—saved by their better-off coreligionists to be held up as a shining example to the rest of Tunis.[60]

The debate over the plans for this utopian project was intense. In the view of those advocating reform, the new construction had to reflect the Jews' status as members of the bourgeois class, or at least a class occupying a middle ground between the colonizers and the Muslim *indigènes*. Through the physical infrastructure of the buildings themselves, the new "European" area would impress on all those who entered it that Tunisian Jews were somehow separate from the "native" people and had cast their lot with the French. Whether the Jews in the hara shared these desires and aspirations was not a concern. Reform-minded Jews, in Paris and in Tunis, had finally found a way—through a powerful combination of Jewish and French prestige and funds—to raise their brethren out of misery and, at the same time, spare themselves the embarrassment of a Saint-Gervais in the colonial setting. In many ways reform of the hara was even more important to French prestige than sanitary intervention in Saint-Gervais. The French government was sensitive about its international reputation. Among the concert of European nations that colonized the world, France touted its imperial presence as a unique gift of French modernity and civilization. Whereas Saint-Gervais could be swept under the rug, in Tunis the all-seeing, ever-critical eye of the empire watched, judged, and evaluated the fitness of its putative citizens. The French and—if they wanted to unite forces with them—the Jews had to emphasize to the Muslim majority the power, status, and opportunity that could be realized through active cooperation with the colonial overlords.

In the early decades of the twentieth century, Tunis was a rapidly expanding city. In 1923 the Tunis Municipal Council commissioned a report to assess the existing infrastructure of the city's buildings and to gauge the level of construction that had taken place over the previous thirty years. The municipal council's report noted the growing value of property in the hands of Tunisian Jews vis-à-vis their Muslim counterparts.[61] In 1923 Jews owned 7 percent of property in Tunis, whereas Muslims owned 71 percent.[62] However, the value of the 7 percent of property owned by Jews represented 14 percent of the total value of property in Tunis; the 71 percent of land owned by Muslims accounted for a mere 30 percent of property value there. These statistics illustrate not only a wide disparity of wealth between Tunisian Jews and Muslims but also a dramatic disparity among Jews themselves. The low property values in the hara (the lowest in Tunis) were more than counterbalanced by the high value of the new construction being done by Jews who were moving into the French sector and suburbs, like La Goulette and La Marsa. Of the seven "essentialized" categories represented in the report, the overall value of the property held by Jews showed the largest increase—a whopping 168 percent growth in land value between 1893 and 1923.[63]

In contrast to the relative lack of concern among Parisian Jews for their coreligionists in Saint-Gervais, bourgeois Parisian Jews actively cooperated with wealthy Tunisian Jews and the colonial government to remedy the plight of indigent Jews in the hara. This difference in attitude is likely the result of two considerations. First, the French were more sensitive to the imperial exigencies of the *mission civilisatrice* than to any moral obligation toward alleviating poverty in their own backyard. It is true that the Comité de Bienfaisance Israélite de Paris, created in 1809, worked assiduously to alleviate the worst suffering of indigent Jews in Paris. However, their resources and power paled in comparison to the capital and clout wielded by the French state. Second, colonial Tunis, in the eyes of Parisian Jews, especially those involved in the AIU's activities, represented a tabula rasa that was suitable for large-scale intervention in a way that was inconceivable in Third Republic Paris. Hence, the primary predicament presented to the Tunis Municipal Council was not whether Jews in the Tunis hara should be "reformed" and rehoused but rather what would be the physical characteristics of this new housing. It was imperative to the council that the new buildings both mold domestic behavior and reflect the bourgeois aspirations of the future inhabitants.

On November 29, 1930, the Tunis Municipal Council, following the recommendations of the SAPH, finalized plans for the demolition, or "cleansing," of the hara—140,000 square meters of land, holding 1,200 buildings.[64] Although the new quarter would ostensibly benefit Tunisian Jews, their cooperation with the expropriation did not progress seamlessly. The Jewish community of Tunis argued that the destruction of the Hobra Synagogue and the Or Thora School, the only school in Tunis dedicated to Talmudic studies, was indefensible. Furthermore, the community contended that it did not possess the necessary funds to rebuild these edifices once they were destroyed. To smooth opposition, the municipal council agreed to cede 400 square meters of land to the community in exchange for the parcels of land occupied by the Hobra Synagogue and the Or Thora School.[65] A similar favorable deal was struck with the Garderie Israélite (Jewish daycare). The Community Council of the Portuguese Jews of Tunis, not wanting to be excluded from the action, claimed that the "normal price" offered by the city for their expropriated land was not sufficient to build a new synagogue for the Grana community. Thus, the city ceded 300 square meters of land to that community. However, when the time came for the demolition of the Hobra Synagogue and the Or Thora School, the community refused to abandon the buildings; they claimed that they still did not possess enough funds to rebuild them. The city, not willing to delay its schemes, caved in to the demands. The municipal council granted the Jewish Community of Tunis an additional 100 square meters of land (500 square meters total) plus parcels of land for the construction of a school and a ritual bathhouse. Furthermore, the buildings would remain tax exempt for the next fifty years.[66] Watching the success of their Jewish brothers, Muslims, in turn, refused to abandon the mosque on the rue de la Margelle that was impeding the construction of the third housing complex. They too claimed that they would not have the necessary funds to rebuild their mosque once it was destroyed. The city grudgingly agreed to grant them 200 square meters on the outskirts of the new quarter, much less space than had been allotted to either community of Jews.[67] Once again, the municipal council let there be no doubt who would be the beneficiaries of the new quarter—indigenous Muslims figured very little in their plans.

Regardless of how the city obtained the land or the price that had to be paid, one thing was clear: the Tunis Municipal Council wanted direct control of all that would be rebuilt in the hara once the expropriations were complete. But micromanaging every detail took its toll. Project design and implementation dragged on, council members squabbled, and funds allotted for the venture evaporated. By the mid-1930s France, which had once lauded itself as impervious to the "American" Great Depression, was beginning to experience a sudden downturn in production and great instability in the value of the franc. As the Tunis Municipal Council demanded increasing funds to build its idyllic Jewish neighborhood, the Grand Council of Tunisia and the resident general, whose decisions the Grand Council rubber-stamped, balked. The Grand Council, which held the purse strings, informed the Municipal Council that the funds would not be forthcoming; the city would have to work out its own solution. The Municipal Council was outraged. City councilman Georges Hignard, appalled that the Grand Council had reneged on the promised funds, complained that the city of Tunis now owned a vast slum and had no money to demolish it, not to mention rebuild it. The Municipal Council, in his view, had become the "vultures of the hara."[68] Some members advocated raising money by selling off the prime real estate slated to surround the newly created square at the Porte de France, as well as property fronting the (never realized) grand avenues that would bisect the hara. Regardless of these schemes, the Municipal Council realized that there would not be enough money to carry out the demolition and reconstruction campaign.

In addition to the recalcitrance of the Grand Council, as the second set of housing units were being completed, the workers went on strike. Tunis was rocked by nationalist unrest and rioting workers, aggravated by inflation, food shortages, and waves of migrant workers fleeing drought in the countryside. The government was forced to concede to various demands of the striking workers, including a pay rise from 1.25 francs to 2 francs per day for each worker and a maximum forty-hour workweek.

Implementation of these measures passed in December 1937–January 1938 caused the hara project to balloon 450,000 francs over budget.[69] The Municipal Council, refusing to agree to any arrangement whereby they would lose control over the project, appealed yet again to the Grand Council for the funds that had been promised. On May 27, 1938, the Grand Council yielded to a decree by the resident general and approved the funds for the hara project to continue.[70] The Municipal Council wasted no time in setting into motion the plans for housing projects five and six, though World War II ultimately halted the efforts.[71]

Idealized Jewish Space

Before the reconstruction of new housing units in the hara even began, debate erupted in the Tunis Municipal Council over the plans for the buildings that would temporarily house those displaced by expropriation and demolition. The proposed temporary housing plan called for a three-story building able to hold about 100 families to be constructed at Bab El-Khadra. Each family would have a one-room apartment of 12–18 square meters; larger families would get two apartments. Every two apartments would be required to share an oven, every four apartments would share toilet facilities, and every six would share a laundry room. The French representative on the Municipal Council, Bernard Sebaut, argued that each apartment should have a separate oven in order to prevent disputes among tenants. However, the director of public works reminded Sebaut that the structures were merely temporary and that most people from the hara cooked on a *canoun* (a small coal-fueled brazier). Councilman Zammit, a Maltese Jew, interjected that outside Tunis (among Jews and Muslims), communal cooking was quite common. However, the French councilman, unable to accept this unorthodox domestic arrangement, argued that "nevertheless . . . there ought to be an oven for each apartment."[72] In the French bourgeois norm, which was to be the new standard for Tunis's Jews, cooking was something done *en famille*, in one's own kitchen, most certainly not in a communal fashion.[73] The refusal of women in the hara to comply with protectorate dictates signals more than ignorance, or even just resistance to authority. "These women were expressing—and enacting—their own local knowledge, their own mores about bodily well-being and cultural integrity."[74] Although the impoverished Jewish women who inhabited the hara were accustomed to its rudimentary conditions, the Tunis Municipal Council insisted that they required all of the bourgeois trappings of European life in order to be comfortable. This newly elaborated difference between native (Muslim) and French space and customs reified the "need for" a Europeanized Jewish quarter. Segregation from the squalor and uncomfortable closeness of the hara was required to re-create the modern French family on "Oriental" soil and to ensure the success of the Jewish regeneration project.[75]

Tunis Municipal Councilman Paul Thiaucourt brought Gallic reason back to the debate by insisting that someone would be appointed to "oversee" the tenants and "enforce discipline" on those who could not agree to equal access of facilities. If, for lack of domestic equipment, Jewish families could not adhere to French bourgeois notions of domesticity and modernity, they would at least be closely monitored to ensure an orderly, controlled access to those facilities that would be available. Furthermore, Thiaucourt noted that the empty lot next to the building should be transformed into a square in which the Jewish children could "frolic." However, Ahmed Ben Arrous, an indigenous Muslim member of the Tunis Municipal Council, had more pressing concerns than frolicking Jewish children; he proposed a similar building be constructed for the needy Muslim community. Thiaucourt, again the self-appointed voice of reason, responded that a building for Muslims had "nothing to do with the hara, which we are currently discussing." Besides, he argued, once the Jews were rehoused in their new buildings in the "European quarter" that was replacing the hara, Muslims could take possession of the abandoned "temporary" housing vacated by the Jews.[76] The ways in which the regime offered solutions to political and social problems through the lens of ethnicity and religion aggravated preexisting tensions between Jews and Muslims, "served to divert attention from the failures of the local French authorities," and provided "justification for the continued concentration of power in their hands."[77]

On November 18, 1935, Dr. Antoine Cassar, a renowned Jewish physician, announced to the municipal council that the temporary housing at Bab El-Khadra was complete; now the real work could begin on construction of the permanent "European-style" housing in the former hara. Cassar reported that because these structures would permanently house the hara's former residents, each apartment would comprise *two* rooms, a small kitchen, and an en suite toilet fit for a "working family."[78] In reality, any "working family" in Paris, not to mention in Tunis, would indeed have been envious of such an apartment. Stores and shops would occupy the first floor of the buildings for the convenience of the tenants. The Municipal Council agreed that tenancy would be reserved exclusively for Jews. Once again, a Muslim councilman, Mohamed el Fourati, beseeched the council, "I discussed with the Commission of Public Works regarding the construction of a building for Muslims who live in the zone that is slated to be demolished, and I would like to know if the Director of Public Works intends to construct a building specific to the usages and customs of Muslims?" The director rebuffed the request, stating, "The first building is intended to house those who were moved out in the first place; when we get to the areas that concern you, we will have new rehousing to think of and at that time we will think about housing specially reserved for Muslims."[79] Apparently, accommodating indigenous Muslims was antithetical to the council's scheme for a "European quarter." To remove any indigenous Muslims who impeded the demolition and reconstruction efforts, on July 29, 1935, the bey, at the behest of Resident General Marcel Peyrouton, had issued a decree that allowed the city of Tunis to expropriate any and all land in the hara "for public utility." This decree freed the council to expropriate hitherto sacrosanct Muslim lands and schools within the prescribed zone.[80] Recalcitrant Muslim landowners could no longer stand in the way of the Municipal Council's vision of a modern, Europeanized Jewish Shangri-la.

Urban housing reform and the travails implicit in its smooth operation serve as an extended metaphor for the modernizing colonial endeavor at large. France—the self-anointed heroine of our story—transports rational science and medicine abroad, quells and civilizes the natives, and brings domestic bliss to traditional, chaotic Oriental space. When contemporary literature, such as that distributed at the Colonial Exposition, deigned to speak of aggressive colonial expansion, exploitation, and domination over indigenous space, it did so with an air of casual disdain for colonial peoples. Reform of social space, domestic norms, and hygienic infrastructure—all rationalized by the authority of science and medicine—operated on an interconnected plane labeled by the French as urban design. Metropolitan France implicitly assumed, and hence legitimated, the importance of imperial domination in maintaining the supremacy of French urban design, which was reflected in, and reified by, urban destruction and creation schemes in the colonies.[81] Ever-evolving economic and political exigencies complicated France's efforts to restructure social space at home; however, a discrete group of Jews assimilated to the cultural authority of France was eager, for the sake of coreligionists, to act out the tenets of French urban design within the confines of the Jewish quarter of Tunis.

In both the metropolitan capital and the colonies, cleansing and reordering urban space took on meanings much more broad than hygienic concern. To be sure, colonial elites were disquieted by what they viewed as the filth and disorder of indigenous space, but hygienic reform also offered colonists a benign, if not altruistic, pretense to reorder and rearrange colonized space according to metropolitan standards—metropolitan standards that were rarely achieved in the metropole. In fact, to justify the intrusive and invasive nature of the spatial reorganization, the bar for hygienic standards was set much higher in the colonies than in the metropole. And nowhere was this concern shown more attention than in consideration of the Jewish quarter. In the French mind, Jewish space in France and the colonies was suspect—a foreign space—and this space, like the Jews that inhabited it, required cleansing and "Frenchification."[82] To the French, Jews were a domestic threat, albeit a familiar one. In spite of the contempt bred by this familiarity, French Christians identified the Jewish community as a fertile point of insertion for French culture and assimilation.

A new generation of urban reformers, such as Henri Prost and Le Corbusier, stymied by the intransigence of French politics at home, tested their ideas for total spatial reorganization in the colonies.[83] Those charged with spatially reorganizing Tunis adhered to the patterns that these young guns, supported by powerful architectural dabblers, like Resident General of Morocco Hubert Lyautey, had established: a new commercial center, or *ville nouvelle,* built according to French standards was constructed contiguous to the "Arab" medina and Kasbah, which would be preserved. Satellite communities, buffered by green spaces (*cordons sanitaires*), were planned around this central urban core. In most of the larger cities in the Maghrib, the Jewish quarters were clearly defined, sometimes walled-in spaces that abutted the medina.[84] Although there was considerable commercial exchange between the Jewish quarters and the rest of the city, everyone recognized the boundaries of each space.

The Tunis Jewish quarter was unique in that it was not an explicitly defined, walled-in space, although it does seem that Jews were confined to its general vicinity until the 1870s.[85] Nevertheless, there were streets in the hara that were predominantly occupied by Muslims or immigrant Maltese and Italian Christians. Although the *tunisois* understood the hara as Jewish space, in reality it was a highly diverse area of metropolitan Tunis, and it was difficult to discern where "Jewish space" left off and the spaces of other ethno-religious groups began. If the map of colonial Tunis is described as a "mosaic" of ethnic neighborhoods, the hara was a mini-melting pot within that mosaic tapestry.[86] Perhaps it was the inability of colonial officials to categorize and define the Tunis hara that led to its demise. In the highly racialized and rigidly structured environment of the French colonies, a neighborhood with a hybrid identity, a zone that existed in an indefinable, liminal space, was intolerable.

By the turn of the nineteenth century, Jews willingly left the Tunis hara as soon as they were financially able to do so. Those Jews who remained in the hara lived with constant social pressure to move their families to a newly created "Jewish suburb" or to the modern *ville nouvelle.* Although Jews began leaving the hara in larger numbers in the late nineteenth century, most Jews left the hara in the shadow of the wrecking ball during the mid- and late 1930s. Regardless of the circumstances under which they left their former homes, the fact is that they did leave. The hara was no longer a Jewish quarter—in fact, by the advent of the Second World War, it no longer existed save for in the memory of those who had once called it home.

Although the French and their assimilated followers had decided that traditional Jews in the hara were ready for their social and moral ascent to French modernity, the eagerness of those in the hara remained less than enthusiastic. In fact, many indigenous Jews harbored their own ideas of modernity that conflicted with those disseminated by the French. Modernity, progress, and regeneration were not concepts to which the French held exclusive rights. Some Tunisian Jews expressed their aspirations for modernity through other avenues, such as Zionism, sports, or theatrical performance, while others resisted and subverted the desire of any "foreign" group to modify their chosen way of life.

The pressures that Frenchified Jews in Paris brought to bear on Jews in Tunisia mirrored similar efforts in the metropole. Paula Hyman has pointed out that a broader idea of Jewishness was developing in Paris during the interwar years with the arrival of eastern Jews. My exploration of these early attempts to create a unified Jewish community in Paris in terms of urban reformation and regeneration sheds new light on the similar transformations that were occurring in colonial space and underscores the impediments to the wholesale adoption of the metropolitan model in Tunis. Although French Jews set out to transform and homogenize the new arrivals, eastern Jews did not accept the notion that acceptance meant turning their backs on their cultural and ethnic roots and deep religious practice. Many of the new arrivals refused to discard their identities, and at the same time, many within French Jewish establishment toyed with the notion that a peaceful symbiosis of "Jewish tradition" and "Frenchness" was possible.[87] In spite of this broadening of the definition of acceptable Jewish comportment, it seems that there was less elasticity in the colonial environment than in metropolitan France regarding the tolerable limits of "foreign expression," and the French establishment, Christians and Jews, consistently underestimated the power of individuals and movements within the Tunisian Jewish community that would resist their efforts to homogenize Jews.

Urban planners in Tunis, as elsewhere in the Maghrib, sought to preserve "authentic" historical space as a living museum of Oriental culture. Scholars have shown how French schemes acted out the colonial policy of "association" in regard to urban reform: on the one hand celebrating the cultural uniqueness of indigenous architecture; on the other, promoting a reorganization of urban space that would advance French interests.[88] It is interesting that, in the case of Tunis, neither the French administration nor the Jews who advocated razing the hara viewed Jewish space as "authentic" or "historical" indigenous space. Somehow the hara did not adequately represent the traditional Orient that the French were seeking to preserve—the same traditional Orient from which assimilated Jews were seeking to shake their brethren free. In other words, in the eyes of the colonial power and their Jewish devotees, the only Maghribi space that could be classified as authentic and historically worthy of preservation bore direct association with Islam, reifying the notion of the static and tradition-bound "Islamic city."

By the early twentieth century, bourgeois reformers deployed sanitary science as an authoritative epistemological weapon in the arsenal of state intervention, and the scientific authority of public health and urban planning provided a fig leaf of evenhandedness to cover the naked zeal of crusaders sent to root out degeneration in the Maghrib. But in the tradition of nineteenth-century positivism, social and political reformers routinely described regeneration in its myriad expressions as the detached, albeit compassionate practice of modern science and medicine. In spite of the trope that "One must follow the same principles of hygiene in the colonies as in France, whether in the city or in the country," the Jewish neighborhoods of Tunis saw far greater hygienic intervention than those of Paris.[89] Only a score of years after the debate over what to do with the Paris ghetto, a similar debate was taking place in the colonies: what should be done with filthy areas of Tunis largely occupied by Jews? In a city with vague expropriation laws, powerless property holders, and willful colonial overlords, the results would be very different indeed. However, the key difference between urban design and sanitary intervention in Paris and Tunis was that the hara of Tunis was destroyed not as a punitive measure, as an economic venture, or for racist motives, but as an effort, primarily spearheaded by Jews, to help *regenerate* their brethren. Ironically, in terms of sanitary and municipal urban reforms, Tunis's Jews experienced the material fruits of French science and medicine before their indigent coreligionists in the imperial capital.

4 Regenerating Youth

The Role of the Alliance and the Rise of Zionism

"Are we not all a little guilty after all? Lazy, because we have so many idlers? Timid, because we let ourselves be oppressed." Willfully created and spread by the colonizer, this mythical and degrading portrait ends up being accepted and lived with to a certain extent by the colonized. It thus acquires a certain amount of reality and contributes to the true portrait of the colonized.

—ALBERT MEMMI, *The Colonizer and the Colonized*

The preceding two chapters have considered how scientific and medical authority defined the parameters of modern and regenerated space. As we have seen, according to this line of thought, the Arab people, as a stagnant race that had been stultified by the limitations of Islam, found a natural home in areas of "historical degeneration," like the central medina or Kasbah. But those who were invested in modernity and the future of French-ruled Tunisia, like the French settlers and their Jewish allies, required state-of-the-art regenerated spaces that mirrored their human potential. In this chapter we turn our attention to that human potential in a more literal sense.

The Jewish body and psyche had long been the object of scientific and medical scrutiny, most of it concluding that Jews were a defective, weak, and ill-formed race. However, the eugenics movement of the late nineteenth and early twentieth centuries gave hope to a new generation of Jews steeped in the promises of regeneration. It was not just physical space that could be ameliorated through regeneration; regeneration also carried the promise of social, cultural, and physical transformation and perfection. This chapter explores how Tunis's Jews understood and interpreted the messages of self-regeneration—an intellectual examination that would ultimately lead to a bifurcation of the community even more dramatic than the rift between Grana and Twansa two centuries earlier.

The early twentieth century was an era of relative peace and upward mobility for Tunisia's Jews. The most important debates of the time questioned definitions of self and community and probed the nature of the relationship between the colonizer and the colonized and among the colonized themselves. Tunisian Jews struggled to define their place in a new Franco-Tunisian colonial society. Two unique strains of "regenerationist" rhetoric—one social and moral, led by the conservative, pro-French forces of the AIU, and the other, physical and muscular, fronted by the vibrant voice of Zionism—divided Tunisian Jewish public opinion in the era between the establishment of the French protectorate (1881) and the onset of World War II.[1]

Again, when I describe the late nineteenth- and early twentieth-century Jewish community of Tunisia, it is with all of the caveats discussed in the introductory chapter. The hitherto divided communities of Twansa and Grana Jews were coalescing into one Tunisian Jewish colonial identity influenced by the call to modernity and a will to regenerate. As this chapter will show, the competing messages of how to achieve regeneration, either through French acculturation or "muscular" Zionism, battled for primacy in this new, loosely amalgamated community of colonial Jews. Regardless of the ideological justification for regeneration, once the effort had begun it was impossible to backtrack to a precolonial identity.

The Alliance Israélite Universelle

The stated purpose of the AIU, founded by Adolphe Crémieux in 1860, was to negotiate with worldwide political authorities on behalf of oppressed

"Oriental Jews" (the catchall term for Jews of the Middle East and North Africa) and to "regenerate" these Jews and prepare them for emancipation via French civilization.[2] The regeneration of wayward Jews into the family of Frenchmen had particular salience in the French Protectorate of Tunisia, where the boundaries between the included and the marginalized were in flux and under constant scrutiny. Eager to not repeat the wholesale naturalization of Jews that had occurred in Algeria in 1870, which they now viewed as a "mistake" that spawned anti-Semitism, French officials in neighboring Tunisia opted for a more selective approach. But exactly how should the regime cherry-pick the desirables from among the masses of socially inept and morally bankrupt Jews, sundry "Arabs" and "Orientals" who claimed rights as equal citizens?

In much the same manner that France utilized the powerful tool of secular republican elementary education to transform her own peasants into Frenchmen, the AIU suggested the social and moral regeneration of backward Oriental Jews via an extensive network of schools dotting the Mediterranean basin. From Iraq to Morocco, the AIU established hundreds of schools centered on the regeneration of Jewish children through exposure to the virtues of French patriotism and "pride in the French language and culture."[3] Just as metropolitan France had weeded the clerics and others hostile to the Republic out of the school system, the effective operation of AIU classrooms as a proving ground for the French civilizing mission hinged on the selection and training of worthy instructors. After all, the brunt of the assignment to save the children of the ghettos would fall on their shoulders. Demonstrating the latent but attainable faculties of moral regeneration, the AIU identified and promoted its instructors from within starting with its very first classrooms in the Near East. These select AIU students who demonstrated the moral and social bearing compatible with the requirements of French civilization were sent to the AIU's Paris training academy, the École Normale Israélite Orientale (ENIO), where they would be transformed into AIU instructors. The new instructors provided living proof to the Jewish communities in France and throughout the diaspora that through exposure to French civilization Oriental Jews could be "made good."

Once settled into the dormitories of the ENIO in Paris, the "little Orientals," as they were called, all dressed uniformly, learned together, and even took walks through the Jardin du Luxembourg as a group, once or twice a week "in single file, chaperoned by one of the teachers."[4] The treatment of these adolescent men and women, who had been uprooted from their friends, families, and familiar surroundings, was both bewildering and infantilizing. Archival records indicate that on one occasion, the Paris staff expressed surprise that the new recruits knew how to eat with forks. In addition to the degrading surveillance and regimental uniformity, the young pupils were repeatedly admonished for their "familiarity."

According to the AIU hierarchy, flamboyance and social impropriety characterized the Oriental Jew, and any such behavior must be nipped in the bud. The AIU administration had made sure to choose well-mannered young men and women with a pleasant physical appearance, a sober demeanor, and no hint of vulgarity, and it was important that they remain this way. The hallmark of ascension to Frenchness was defined by the acceptance and practice of "good manners," and through the mastery of correct social behavior, the "little Orientals" proved their conquest over innate barbarism.[5]

Once trained, AIU instructors were sent out to new schools springing up throughout the Mediterranean basin and Near East, including Tunisia. Between 1878 and 1910, the AIU founded three schools for boys and one for girls in Tunis. Malta Srira for boys was the first. The AIU also opened schools in other Tunisian cities: Sousse had a school for boys founded in 1883, and Sfax had one school for boys and one for girls founded in 1905. From their inception, alliance schools in Tunisia were very popular. Over a thousand students enrolled in the inaugural year, 1878. By 1913 there were well over three thousand students enrolled in alliance schools in Tunisia.[6]

As for the curriculum, alliance classrooms focused on fluency in French language (most students in Tunisia spoke Judeo-Arabic at home). Once the French language had been mastered, the pupils conquered French literature and history. Using French textbooks, including *Our Ancestors: The Gauls*, Tunisian Jews were trained in ersatz French republican classrooms. Class walls were plastered with maps of France and adorned with the portrait of the president of the French Republic—there was little or no reference to the local region. Added to this French curriculum, the pedagogical ethos closely mimicked the French system on which it was modeled. Students learned by rote, instructors were domineering and distant, and inculcation was often more punitive than edifying. Instructors expected children, treated as miniature adults, to work diligently in rather uncomfortable, joyless, and Spartan surroundings.

As had been the case at the ENIO, Paris officials frowned on emotional closeness; camaraderie between students and between students and instructors was discouraged. One roving AIU supervisor complained in a letter to Paris headquarters, "Mr. Benbassat [an alliance director in Tunis] uses the familiar *tu* but also calls him [a fellow alliance instructor] 'Loria' in front of his students. Mr. Loria follows this lead. This is bad both for the director's prestige and for discipline in the school in general. I made a point of discussing this issue with Mr. Loria."[7] In their correspondence with the Paris administration, AIU instructors repeatedly bemoaned the squalor of the Tunis Jewish ghetto (hara) and, more important, the "degenerated" state of Jewish children. In a series of letters written by alliance instructor L. Guéron from Tunis to central headquarters in Paris, Guéron noted that although the alliance had been present at that time for more than thirty years in Tunis, Jews in the hara remained "thick and fleshy" and "arthritic or neurasthenic." To rectify these evils, Guéron recommended that hara Jews embrace a "love of physical cleanliness" and "a good amount of well-directed physical exercise."[8] In spite of the suggestions from Guéron and other instructors that healthy exercise should be incorporated into the daily routine as a complement to social and moral regeneration, young children in alliance schools were allotted no time for physical education, and older children received a scant maximum of two hours of physical education per week.[9] The AIU was doing little to harness the physical energy and enthusiasm of its pupils.

As the AIU continued to harp on the importance of moral and social regeneration, the ideological construction and philosophical underpinnings of the regeneration movement within the scientific community began to take more of a "physical," biomedical turn. Buttressed by the emergence of "race science," regeneration was now viewed as not just a social and moral undertaking but also a scientific quest to enhance the physical "fitness" of the species. There is little doubt that metropolitan France was anxious about degeneration, especially in light of "the defeat" in 1870 and the decadence of the Belle Époque. Hence, the public "reacted favorably to a 'hygienic' physical culture that promised some hope of national regeneration" in light of the "deepening sense of anxiety about the biological health of the national stock."[10] Although Darwinian evolutionary theory, as an overarching concept, was relatively well received in France, many authorities maintained that natural selection was not the catalyst for evolutionary adaptation.[11] The predominant view in France was that humans were capable of improving their mind, culture, and body and those who ameliorated their "fitness" could pass biological advantages on to their children. The natural converse of this theory was that deleterious characteristics acquired through years of vicious behavior and brutish living conditions became dominant traits—the *medical* disorder of degeneration—that could likewise be transmitted to offspring.[12]

Although it can be argued that these Lamarckian (and later neo-Lamarckian) interpretations of the heritability of acquired traits reigned in France well into the early twentieth century, long after other European nations and the United States had embraced Mendelian inheritance, it is also true that conceptions of race and trait heritability were fluid and, even within the French scientific community, highly contested.[13] Although the French did lag in their acceptance of Mendelian heritability, Lamarckian conceptions of adaptation, trait heritability, and racial hierarchy likely had just as much to do with the maintenance of the socioeconomic status quo and justifications for colonial domination as with a consensus view within the French scientific community. Ideas of heritability, racial stock, and degeneration were important in metropolitan France, but they were compellingly salient in the French colonies, where such ideas offered rational, scientific explanations for indigenous backwardness and further justification for French domination, intervention, and paternalism.[14]

Numerous works in Jewish studies detail the obsessive dedication with which Western medical authorities (including Jews) described the physical and moral unfitness of ghetto-dwelling Jews and the way, over time, the resolute power of Western medical discourse and science reinforced the widely accepted view of Jews as pathologized subjects, racially and biomedically unfit.[15] The Jewish community held a unique position in that it was a discrete "racial" group with both a metropolitan and colonial constituency. Moreover, Jewish scientists, physicians, and philosophers were also part of the broader European academic community that diligently undertook the task of classifying and ranking humanity. While this racialized language interjected with scientific credibility gave ready fodder, in the French context, to anti-Semites like Georges Vacher de Lapouge and Edouard Drumont, it also provided powerful discursive legitimacy to the emerging Zionist movement, which relied heavily on the biological metaphors of hygiene, fitness, purity, and physical regeneration.[16]

Zionism and Muscular Judaism

With modern science in mind, the growing Zionist movement offered its own antidote to the physical and moral decay of Jews. Muscular Judaism, as the movement came to be called, was a political and hygiene movement that sought to revive the past glory and strength of the Jewish people through physical activity, often combined with renewed contacts with rural life.[17] The regenerated Jewish body exemplified by this movement defied common stereotypes of the ghetto-dwelling Jew, bound to a designated space, profession, and mode of life.

> Whereas eugenics aspired to redeem the human species by forcing it to face the realities of its biological nature, Zionism aspired to redeem the Jewish people by forcing it to face the realities of its biological existence. The Zionists claimed that Jews maintained their ancient distinct "racial" identity, and that their regrouping as a nation in their homeland would have profound eugenic consequences, primarily halting the degeneration they fell prey to because of the conditions imposed on them in the past. Some Zionists believed in

a Lamarckian driven eugenics that expected the "normalization" of Jewish life styles to change their constitution.[18]

Max Nordau and Theodor Herzl disseminated much of this rhetoric, especially as it related to the German context, in their efforts to popularize Zionism.[19] But the image of Jews as stalwart, rational beings who could control their own destiny held wide appeal not just in German-speaking lands. French Jews, influenced by the First World Zionist Congress in Basel (1897), became more attuned to the potential power of the bold Zionist message, especially in the wake of rising anti-Semitism sparked by the Dreyfus Affair.

As the Dreyfus Affair spread its scourge throughout France and the French Empire, many Jews sought a means to counter the anti-Semitic narrative.[20] In reaction to the foundation of the anti-Semitic newspaper *L'Echo Tunisien*, which expressed an anti-Dreyfusard, pro-*colon* point of view, Tunisian Jew Gabriel Allouche organized a well-received conference on "Le Sionisme et les Juifs de Tunisie" in 1897.[21] In spite of the failure to launch a Zionist organization from the conference, Zionism became increasingly visible in the more than fifty Jewish newspapers available to Tunisian Jews by the beginning of the twentieth century. For the most part, these newspapers reported on activities of the Zionist conference and offered news updates from Palestine.[22] As an official arm of the French administration, the AIU had little to say in regard to French anti-Semitism and feared being perceived as apologists for the regime's excesses. But where the AIU remained uncomfortably silent, the newly emerging Zionist movement mounted a vocal opposition. Tunisian Jews found common cause with those demanding human rights and dignity. As subjects of the bey, most Tunisian Jews recognized that the political and judicial structure of the protectorate denied Jews their de facto and de jure civil rights.

During the interwar years, the Zionist movement in Tunisia, mimicking those elsewhere, grew more powerful and splintered into four main groups that have been the subject of much academic attention: the General Zionists, the right-wing Revisionists, the conservative Mizrahi, and the leftist Labor Zionists.[23] The early, less ideologically based Zionist groups that sprouted up during World War I are often termed "general Zionism."[24] General Zionists, also called Synthetic Zionists, embraced all classes and political parties and concentrated on their stated goal of the establishment of Palestine as homeland and refuge for persecuted Jews. However, once the Balfour Declaration of 1917 dangled the possibility of transforming hope into reality, Zionism split into rival groups increasingly based on political and social ideologies. The Revisionists, led by the firebrand Ze'ev Vladimir Jabotinsky, rejected the "accommodationist" strategy of the General Zionists for land acquisition in Palestine and advocated a militant, "pure" approach that refused compromise with both Great Britain and Arab-Palestinians for Palestinian territory. In 1925 Alfred Valensi, the original advocate of General Zionism in Tunisia, defected from the movement and backed the Revisionists, greatly strengthening their position in Tunisia. The primary aim of the ultranationalist Mizrahi Zionists, as voiced in the newspaper, *L'Oeuvre Israélite*, was the rejection of any assimilation to French secularism and an emphasis on religious piety. The final group, the Labor Zionists, founded by Victor Nataf in 1924, advocated freedom from both the oppression of French and Arab nationalists and "oppressive capitalism."[25] The Labor newspaper *La Revue Israélite* and the rival Revisionists newspapers *La Voix d'Israël* and *Le Réveil Juif* conducted a bitter debate for the hearts and minds of the Jewish community that lasted throughout the interwar years.[26]

At first, Zionism in Tunisia was not a community-wide phenomenon; it centered on an elite group of Grana Jews who viewed Zionism as a means to connect with Jewish communities in Europe.[27] In 1911 the lawyer Alfred Valensi officially founded the first Zionist group in Tunisia, Aghoudat Sion, which was linked through the French Zionist Federation (Federation Sioniste Française) to the Zionist Organization (Organisation Sioniste). Valensi published the French-language newspaper associated with the group, *La voix de Sion* (The voice of Zion), which was also translated and published in Judeo-Arabic by Jacob Boccara. However, for most Jews in Tunisia, regardless of class or community—rich or poor, Twansa or Grana—early Zionism had very little to do with identity formation or what we would now call "identity politics." Zionism was more an outward expression of concern for Jewish brethren in distant lands who faced persecution or a method of contact with the European Jewish community. Zionism at this time in Tunisia was a nascent movement that expressed concern for oppressed Jews in Eastern Europe, Russia, and Palestine. In many ways Tunisian Zionism built on the foundation of the Tunisian Haskalah movement led by Rabbi Shalom Flāḥ and expressed in the *Hatzfira* newspaper that he published in the late nineteenth century.[28] The Haskalah movement's goal of Jewish scholarly tradition combined with the values of modernity—a Hebrew Enlightenment—fit well into the early Zionist message of budding Jewish pride and awareness. The AIU, although it fought Zionism at every turn, ironically shared similar goals: a transnational Jewish identity and the modernization of Jews through a celebration and revival of past glory.[29]

But regardless of the brand of Zionism to which a Jew subscribed (or not), by the early 1920s many Tunisian Jews felt caught up in a cultural tug-of-war, displeasing to and suspected by both the French and their fellow Tunisians. The French accused Jews of clinging to their Oriental ways; Tunisian Muslims alleged that Jews did not consider themselves "Tunisian" and only wished to remain Tunisian if protégés of the French government. According to Muslims, Tunisian Jews had been more "Tunisian" before the arrival of the French, and this claim was likely true in many ways. But there were also rifts developing within the Tunisian Jewish community itself. The growing popularity of the Zionist message further complicated the all-consuming debate over the Jew's "proper place"—politically, socially, and culturally.

Before World War II Zionism, as expressed throughout much of Europe and Russia, supported the foundation of a Jewish homeland as a haven for persecuted Jews—Jews could be assured political, social, and judicial equality only within a Jewish homeland. Many French Jews who subscribed to Zionism agreed with this premise, but with an important caveat. Being that French Jews, in their view, were not *persecuted*, they had no need to avail themselves of a Jewish refuge or homeland. French Jews believed that the blood spilt during the French Revolution had guaranteed their political, social, and legal equality. As French citizens, they shared the same rights and obligations as French Christians and displayed a steadfast devotion to Mother France. French acculturated Tunisian Jews, backed by the AIU in Paris, agreed that their path toward equality also lay in full accession to the rights and guarantees of *French* citizenship.

The debate over Tunisian Jewish allegiance vividly played out in the pages of the Jewish press during the interwar years. Jewish news outlets that advocated Revisionist Zionism, such as *La Voix d'Israël* and *Réveil Juif*, launched bitter attacks on the pro-AIU assimilationist newspaper *La Justice*. The rhetorical salvos were returned with vigor, and the community struggled to reconcile the various definitions of Tunisian Jewishness. *La Justice* proclaimed, "God forbid we ever forget to recognize the generous tolerance and hospitality that Tunisia has shown to our ancestors . . . but Tunisia has never been our homeland."[30] However, in lieu of establishing their own Jewish homeland as advocated by the Revisionists, *La Justice* and its followers claimed that their homeland was neither Tunisia nor Palestine, but France.

The protectorate regime doggedly reinforced the message that the correct path to political and judicial equality for Jews was through "Frenchness." In March 1922 the secretary general of Tunisia received a note from a secret informant stating that a Jerban Rabbi, while passing through Tunis, disparaged the AIU for overemphasizing the French language to the detriment of Hebrew.[31] Neither the alliance nor the French administrative apparatus had been able to penetrate Jerba.[32] French officials recognized the internal threat posed by what it deemed to be noncooperative Jews and "traditional" Zionists. The French considered the AIU as an official arm of the French education system and vigorously defended its role in the Jewish community. French officials, and many at the alliance, suspected any educational facility established in the name of the Jewish *religion* or the Hebrew language of harboring a hotbed of Revisionist radicals.

The Palestine riots of 1929 marked a turning point in the relations among Jews, Muslims, and the French regime in Tunisia.[33] Hitherto, Zionists had for the most part governed their functions with the tacit approval of the regime and were largely ignored by the Muslim population. However, in March 1932, under mounting pressure from the Destour Party and the

French security apparatus, the regime cancelled an imminent visit to Tunisia by the radical Revisionist Jabotinsky. To calm the tension, representatives of the Jewish community assured French officials that talk of Zionism would be more "discreet."

The regime also took offense to less ardent Zionist organizations, like Keren Ha-yesod. Whereas French officials and some Tunisian Muslims were more than happy to maintain, and at times exacerbate, the tensions and divisions within the Jewish community to their own aims, Keren Ha-yesod (the Foundation Fund), which had been established at the World Zionist Conference in London in 1920 to raise fund for the establishment of a Jewish settlement in Palestine, preached the unification of all Jews, Zionist and non-Zionist, regardless of nationality or political affiliation in one Jewish homeland. This organization, which welcomed all Jews under a broad nationalist-inspired umbrella, imperiled a regime that advocated assimilation and frowned on the desire for a Jewish homeland. It also challenged the indigenous Muslim narrative of what constituted Tunisian identity. In spite of this disapproval, or perhaps because of it, Jews responded with a vociferous public demonstration in support of Zionism, but also in support of freedom of speech and expression.[34]

In June 1932 Nathan Halpern, the leader of the francophone branch of Keren Ha-yesod, planned a public screening of the film *La Terre Promise* in Tunis. Much to thc chagrin of the Jewish community, French officials refused to allow the screening to go forward, which sparked mass demonstrations for freedom of expression and assembly.[35]

According to the French regime, Keren Ha-yesod posed an existential threat to the stability of the Jewish-Muslim status quo within the protectorate. The mere contemplation of a Jewish identity beyond the parameters of Frenchness was tantamount to radical revisionism.

AIU versus Zionism

In June 1935 Jews in Béja requested permission from French officials to open a Talmud Torah to teach Hebrew to indigent Jewish children. French officials objected to what they saw as the burgeoning power of these Zionist offshoots that poached students from French secular schools and their AIU ally. Alliance officials also feared the proliferation of "traditional" Jewish schools to the detriment of the alliance's more "Western" approach. Those advocating the Talmud Torah tried to allay suspicions by stressing that their school would shelter the children of Béja from the danger and temptations of the streets, especially during vacation. But in a more important concession to gain official approval, the school agreed to impart on their students the "rudiments of [French] family and civic morality."[36] The École Franco-Hebraïque Or Thora, which had existed since 1885, faced a similar struggle to gain official recognition as an elementary school in May 1936. Once again, the sticking point was that the French government wanted reassurance that French would be the primary language of instruction, although the stated purpose of the school was to promote the "vulgarization of the Hebrew language."[37]

In the first part of the twentieth century, as Hebrew grew in use from a textually based religious language into an actual means of daily communication, perception of the language itself changed. The AIU taught "religious Hebrew" but was frightened by the overtly Revisionist implications of teaching Hebrew as a modern "living" language. There was a palpable tension at alliance headquarters in Paris between agreeing to teach Hebrew in order to compete with religious Jewish schools and accepting Hebrew as a language whose importance was on par with French. In the late nineteenth century, the alliance argued that although the Hebrew language had a venerable two-thousand-year history, it was "impractical for the assimilation and comprehension of modern civilization."[38] The alliance admitted that Zionists should continue the development of Hebrew but maintained that pushing Hebrew on students could compromise their future. The alliance argued that Hebrew was not practical as a survival tool in the modern world and "people cannot live on sentiment. One must win his daily bread to survive."[39] By 1913 the AIU entertained the notion of teaching Hebrew in alliance schools. However, some within the alliance cautioned, "Pedagogues affirm that the study of multiple languages is detrimental to the normal development of the child's mental faculties by putting too much strain on a frail body and inhibiting the regular growth of its organs. . . . We are now putting the brains of our young children through intellectual gymnastics to which they are not at all accustomed after several centuries of absolute repose." Teaching children too many languages diluted their ability to express logic and abstract ideas with "intellectual vigor."[40] In other words, pushing the agenda of Hebrew, in the place of French, was not only detrimental to the future economic success of students; it could harm them physically and emotionally.

Similarly, any perceived refusal of French secular education (the French considered the AIU as "Jewish secular") in favor of a religious-based education sent up a red flag for the protectorate. Officials in the French administration and the alliance hierarchy expressed a particular horror of the Talmud Torah, whose students they described as "weak, scrawny, puny, one would say almost ghostlike. . . . Their clothing is generally in rags. Many are barefoot . . . unclean and unkempt."[41] French officials considered these schools, which excluded girls and focused on recitation of the Scriptures and the Talmud in Hebrew, to be counter to the Franco-centric, secular-based education as offered by the AIU, which could combat Jewish backwardness and superstition. The alliance, and officials in the French protectorate, claimed that these children were intellectually capable of expanding beyond the Oriental confines of their surroundings but that the filth and chaos in the Talmud Torah would inevitably hold them back and prevent their full assimilation. Alliance leaders were appalled by the filthiness of the teaching conditions, as well as the paralyzing lack of structure and order. "There is no roll call; no one is marked present or late. The class is noisy. The children get up or sit down, leave or return, talk or remain silent, all under the eyes of the instructors who take no mind of them. It is total disorder."[42]

Emphasizing the distance between "traditional Jewish" disorder and Gallic reason, French officials remained hostile to any effort by Jews to find community outside the rigid framework of cooperative "assimilation" to the French way of life. In October 1935 the secretary general of Tunisia received a request from a group of Jews wishing to form a group called Friends of the Jews in Tunisia. Considering the potential threat of these noncooperative Jews, the French administration balked, stating in a letter transmitted back to the putative organization that organizations of a religious, cultural, and charitable nature were "over-abundant" in the Jewish community in Tunisia. Jews, the secretary general advised, would be better served by focusing their energies on participating in the "official community"—in other words, the French secular community. It is particularly telling that in the original handwritten copy of the letter, the words "legal community" are stricken and replaced with the words "official community."[43] From the non-redacted version, one could infer alternative meanings. Perhaps the French believed that Tunisian Jews tended to find their locus of organization "illegally" and counter to the "community" at large, or the French balked a priori at the notion of considering Jews as a "legal" part of their community. Regardless, these archival records make clear that the French demanded allegiance and adoption of their "civilization," even if they had no clear willingness to accept Tunisian Jews as Frenchmen and equals.

Where acculturated Jews found it difficult to express themselves outside the narrow channels approved by the French authorities, Zionists made inroads. Zionists became more and more adept at couching their rhetoric in the language of youth, corporeal fitness, and progressive, scientific materialism. One AIU instructor described a Zionist meeting in which the local Zionist leader presented "figures, technical information, tables, charts, and schematics through which he demonstrated that Jewish nationalism, according to *modern science*, must take precedent over patriotism; the nationalist ideal, according to *pedagogical science*," must serve as the Jew's guide. Zionists spoke a language that "bristled with science . . . psychology, psycho-physiology, psychiatry, biomechanics, and biochemistry." According to the alliance instructor who witnessed the meeting, "No one really followed what he [the Zionist leader] was saying; so he must have been correct."[44] In spite of the alliance instructor's misgivings, the Zionist message, saturated with modernity, progressive science, and muscular self-assertiveness, resonated strongly with young Jews, especially those of modest means living in the ghetto. The Zionist monthly *Die Jüdische Turnzeitung* (The Jewish gymnastics journal) exhorted, "The one-sided education of the mind, which caused our nervousness and mental fatigue, is what we are fighting! We want to give the limpid Jewish body back its lost vigor, to make it fresh and robust, agile and strong. We want to achieve this in a Jewish association, so that at the same time we can strengthen our unity and raise our self-consciousness, two things that have been dwindling."[45] Apparently, the AIU was not the Jewish association the journal had in mind.

Although the AIU advocated a measured and moderate approach toward Zionism, the alliance recognized that more and more Jews, especially youth, were attracted by the verve of the Zionist message in "this century of outrageous mechanization and materialism."[46] Among the local population, alliance instructors personified Gallicism, assimilation, a refusal of the "Oriental" lifestyle, and most important, a bulwark against Zionism. Compared to the youthfulness and excitement of Zionism, the alliance's path appeared dull and stodgy. And to young children, used to running amok in the Tunis ghetto, the rigid moral inculcation of the alliance instructors must have seemed harsh indeed. It was not just in Tunisia that the Zionists presented themselves as the vigorous, muscular alternative to the AIU's shopworn assimilationist message. An alliance instructor in Turkey also confessed to fear the "pointed red beard, furious eyes, and well-muscled arms" of the leader of the Maccabi sports club.[47] The imagery of "sports and struggle" evoked a pride within Jewish youth that the alliance was unable to duplicate.

But it is clear that Jewish youth, newly empowered by Zionist muscular rhetoric, were becoming more and more content to express themselves as Jews, not French Israelites. In October 1931 all of Tunisia celebrated as Victor "Young" Perez defeated American Frankie Genaro in a second-round knockout and captured the title of Flyweight Champion of the World. Young Perez, a twenty-one-year-old product of the Tunis Jewish ghetto, was an unlikely hero. Zionists were especially proud of the hometown boy and reveled in his success. The explosion of excitement and pride in the Jewish community in Tunis showed that there was a new "type" of Jew on the stage—a "muscular," proud Jew.[48]

In early 1934 *L'Aurore*, the weekly newspaper in Tunisia for "Jewish information and Zionist action," reported on Young Perez's match against French champion Eugène Huat. Huat bragged before the match that Perez feared him "because he knows I am stronger than he is." However, the *L'Aurore* reporter crowed, "As soon as the bell announced the first round, like a tiger on his prey, the 'child of the souks' lunged at his opponent and riddled him with his fists. Under the powerful dynamism of the valorous Tunisian, Huat was momentarily stunned; realizing the value of his adversary."[49] Perhaps the reason why Tunisian Jews celebrated Perez's victory to such a degree was that he defied all common stereotypes of the Tunisian Jew of the hara. He also embodied the success of the physical regeneration efforts promoted from within the Jewish community itself. Although the AIU had turned out many successful former students who had made their way in the world thanks to "moral and behavioral regeneration," none aroused excitement and fervor like the boy who had achieved success and thrilled Tunisia on account of his muscular strength. The Jewish community was now able to express its aggressions through "its" boxer and his victory could be symbolically claimed by the masses that he represented.[50]

In a telling letter to the Quai d'Orsay, the delegate to the resident general complained about the militantly independent nature of this "new" Tunisian Jewish youth.

> Excellent athletes, intrepid runners, boxers who fear none of the inherent risks of the sport, swimmers whose prowess I have recently admired, they [Tunisian Jewish youth] are completely devoid of the timidity . . . *of their ancestors*. Proud of their training, their attitude during these troubled times is openly provocative and reading newspapers like *Le Reveil Juif* that follow a clear Zionist bent, doesn't exactly calm tensions. Every Saturday and Sunday, for nine months of the year, the stadiums of the Tunis suburbs are filled with crowds who have come to see matches between Jews and Italians. . . . These crowds are often so boisterous that the Superior Committee for Sports has had to prevent certain matches between Jews and Italians or Jews and Arabs.[51]

The author makes no mention of the tensions that must have existed between the Jews, "Arabs," and Italians on one side and their colonial French masters on the other. However, letters in the AIU archives indicate that instructors noticed the rivalry between French and Jewish, "Arab," and Italian children on the playing fields. When left to their own devices, the children naturally divided along ethnic and religious lines—Jews often separating off qua Jews. In one such encounter that took place in 1937, Gilbert Chikly recalls that an AIU instructor, Mr. Lara, halted an after-school football match and questioned the composition of the teams. "Mohammed, what are the teams? Who is playing whom?" Mohammed responded, "It's the Arabs against the Jews, sir, a great match up, Halfaouine against the Hara." Mr. Lara furiously called a halt to the match, exclaiming, "Stop! Stop the match and give me the ball. You have no shame; you couldn't find another way to form up teams? Jews against Arabs? You kids are crazy, it's disgusting!" Mr. Lara recomposed each team requiring five Jews and five Arabs on each side.[52] It is difficult to discern the motivation of the students' self-segregation. Was it merely an innocent neighborhood rivalry, or did it represent a more complex, ethno-religious struggle for self-identity? In any case, it is difficult to know if the Jewish boys formed a team as Zionist Jews or as Frenchmen, but one thing is clear—they saw themselves as something other than "Arab Jews."

Alliance instructors in Tunis made a concerted effort to thwart the message of Zionism and urged their students to turn away from political engagement. Alliance instructors admonished Tunisian Jews that "the first duty of a Jew is to be a 'good citizen,' worthy of the country in which he lives and worthy of his glorious heritage."[53] The issue for Tunisian Jews was not a matter of being a "good citizen." It was a deeper question: to whom would this citizenry pledge allegiance—France, Tunisia, or fellow Jews? On the eve of the Second World War, a nascent movement in Tunisia began to seek a social and political identity as something other than French, and perhaps, something other than Tunisian. The German occupation of France and Tunisia and Vichy France's collaboration intensified the call for a Jewish identity independent of either France or Tunisia. In the power vacuum, the muscular and self-reliant voice of Zionism, which had gained social currency and political strength throughout the interwar years, captured the imagination of many of Tunisia's Jews.

During the interwar years, the Tunisian Jewish community further splintered into subgroups according to various social, political, and ethnic criteria, which resulted in a complex array of polyvalent and overlapping interests. For example, although the AIU was explicitly, as an organization, anti-Zionist, there were teachers among the rank and file who sympathized with and participated in Zionism of all stripes. On the other hand, there were alliance teachers who agreed with their leaders and considered Zionism a direct affront to the French *mission civilisatrice*. Similarly, there were fervent Mizrahi Zionists who embraced the French language and civilization. There were also pious Jews who were part of the Labor Zionists and secular Jews who were Revisionists. In short, political, social, religious, and class differences fragmented the Jewish community along lines that were not necessarily predictors of group identity. Local conditions, like the anti-Jewish Sfax riots of 1932, and political realities, like the rise of organized labor and the *Front populaire* in 1936, also influenced group identity as Jews banded together in new ways along shifting historical fault lines.[54] The historical picture is complex and messy. Individual actors often defy categorization by siding with groups opposed to their "rational interests" or by embracing and melding together seemingly competing ideologies. The Tunisian Jewish colonial community was no exception. The chief disagreement concerned who would be the most effective architect of Jewish regeneration. Nevertheless, the direct appeal to the cultural authority of science and medicine and its explicit links to the regeneration of the Jewish people undergirded both AIU and Zionist propaganda.

5 Regenerating Women

The Assertion of Reproductive Control

The fruit is not an accident or miracle of a plant but a sign of its maturity.

— ALBERT MEMMI, *The Colonizer and the Colonized*

Marguerite "Habiba" M'sika was born in the Jewish ghetto of Tunis in 1903 to a family of impoverished string merchants. Like many indigent Jewish girls in Tunis, Marguerite attended school at the French-led AIU, where she spent seven years learning to read, write, and master various skills, such as sewing and handicrafts, that would mold her into a proper French lady. But in spite of the careful inculcation of the alliance instructors, Marguerite had ideas of her own.[1] In her early teens, she left the alliance and began to spend more time with her songstress aunt who ran the local *bain maure* (Moorish bath, hammam). Adopting the pseudonym "Habiba" (beloved), the young girl began to train as a singer, dancer, and actor under the tutelage of her aunt and practice her charms on the hammam's clientele. By the early 1920s Habiba's fame and notoriety had spread—she had become a star and, perhaps, the first sex symbol in Tunisian history. Although married to her cousin, she carried on numerous affairs with French, Jewish, and Muslim notables.

Followed around Tunis by her band of loyal male fans that called themselves "soldiers of the night" (*asakir al-lil*), Habiba flitted from performance to performance collecting more fans and even more lovers. In 1925 Habiba scandalized Tunis when she was cast as Romeo in the production of *Romeo and Juliet*. The onstage kiss between Romeo and her fellow female actress, Juliet, provoked an outrage that could be broken up only by Habiba's loyal "soldiers," who set fire to the stage in executing her rescue and escape from the theatrical venue.

While carrying on yet another scandalous affair, this time with Prince Fuad of Egypt, Habiba met Eliahou Mimouni, an elderly Jew from Testour, Tunisia. As was her nature, Habiba fanned the flames of Mimouni's desperate infatuation. Mimouni built a palace for her and begged her to become his lover. When Habiba rebuffed his advances, on February 20, 1930, Mimouni sneaked into Habiba's apartment in Tunis, doused her in gasoline, and set her on fire. The following day, Mimouni sat vigil at Habiba's hospital beside as she slid into a coma and died. Habiba M'sika's funeral procession is recorded as one of the largest in Tunisian history, rivaling that of President Habib Bourguiba.

Beyond the fascinating tale of her meteoric rise to fame and horrifically tragic death, what can we, as historians, glean from Habiba's universal allure? What was it about her that made her so captivating to interwar-era Tunisians and present-day observers alike? Taken in isolation, the life of Habiba recounts the oft-told tale of an overly ambitious courtesan or showgirl—a *provocateuse*. But in a larger sense, her flamboyant zest for life vividly demonstrates the social and cultural power of modernity in colonial life. Whether adored or reviled, all agreed on one point: Habiba was modern. Her tale exemplifies the dichotomous nature inherent in "living colonialism," walking the tightrope between modern and indigenous, liberated and subjugated, and civilized and native. More important, her story reflects the tension within the Jewish community in regard to the proper role of women and their place in a modern society. Embracing French modernity, if that is indeed what Habiba represented, and the emancipation of women upended indigenous cultural and religious norms. As the lynchpin to regeneration, women and, even more important, their reproductive powers lay at the heart of successful colonial assimilationist policy. Novel medical interventions and lifesaving technologies, especially in regard to childbirth, attracted Tunisian Jewish women, but the acceptance of French medicine and scientific expertise also implied a rejection of indigenous traditions. Ordinary Jewish women were forced to walk the same tightrope as Habiba. Jewish women balanced indigenous practices with French medicine, melded native understandings with scientific savoir faire, and renegotiated their subjugated status into liberated womanhood. For Tunisian Jewish women, embracing French medicine and science was simultaneously a cultural imposition and a positive outgrowth of colonialism.

Demonstrations of modernity through scientific advancement, medical skill, and technological prowess were key indications of the successful regeneration of colonial men. But where women were concerned, both in the metropole and the colonies, modernity was a double-edged sword, often labeled as a luxurious and petulant whim for freedom, feminism, and childlessness that more often than not opened the door to the degeneration of the race, not its renaissance. According to this line of thought, men demonstrated their modernity through the assimilation of intellectual and technological precepts; women flouted their modernity through unorthodox, outlandish behavior. Of course, careful examination of the historical record disabuses us of this overly simplistic reduction.

Habiba's contemporary critics claimed that she embodied all that was degenerative, decadent, and dangerous about the expression of colonial modernity in women. But not every woman could be, or wanted to be, the next Habiba. Habiba was feted and scorned by Tunisian society because she was an outlier and an anomaly. The majority of women asserted their role as regenerators, and progenitors, through a determined effort to maintain control of their bodies and reproduction against the growing trends to medicalize and pathologize the female body and relocate childbirth to the clinical setting.

Much has been written regarding the medicalization of society in Western Europe and the United States in the modern era. Eager to name, classify, and obsessively describe pathologies, as well as natural physiological occurrences, such as pregnancy and childbirth, physicians and public health officials elaborated new fields of medicine dedicated to the hygienic and scientific management of these bodily functions. Physiological knowledge, as constructed by learned medical men, had long considered the female body as mysterious but also prone to innate weakness, demonic possession, and illness.[2] Intensive investigation of the female anatomy by male physicians, instead of dispelling the mythologies of "female problems," tended to reify and ascribe scientific nomenclature to the supposed defective traits and functions of the female body.

In the late nineteenth and early twentieth centuries, Western scientists made medical and laboratory discoveries that would forever alter our perception of the human body and its pathologies. These revolutionary changes, which have been described by various historians of medicine as the "rise of scientific authority," the "therapeutic revolution," and the "social transformation" of medicine changed not only the ways in which physicians understood the body; they also further alienated laypeople from understanding their own sickness and health.[3] Part of these revolutionary changes manifested themselves through a newfound preoccupation of scientists and doctors with the welfare of mothers and infants, in part owing to the validation of these subjects as worthy of examination by the medical establishment. In the final decades of the nineteenth century, the medical community essayed to appropriate and redefine reproductive science and child rearing as skills that required scientific knowledge and medical training. Obstetrics, gynecology, and pediatrics became recognized as male-dominated fields with attendant journals, professional societies, and prescribed university coursework.

This chapter investigates the social, economic, and cultural aspects of medicalized maternity in the Jewish community of French colonial Tunis in the late nineteenth and early twentieth centuries. It explores the ramifications of the adoption of "germ conscious" practices by Jewish mothers and homemakers. It also examines the ways in which the purported triumph of medical expertise and scientific knowledge shaped future social relations, perceptions, and practices among Jewish mothers in Tunis and functioned as a powerful tool of acculturation to French bourgeois norms. Upper-echelon, French-acculturated Jewish women preached the "gospel of germs" and its message of normative, bourgeois conformity to working-class, "Arab" Jews and used female charitable networks to disseminate "modern" hygienic practices and nutritional advice beyond a scope accessible to "outside" male physicians.[4]

On the surface the medicalization of childbirth and motherhood reified male domination over female bodies, but it was also a means by which women could harness the powerful rhetoric of national identity creation. Now, women could be instructed—and instruct other women—on proper mothering techniques and the inculcation of skills specific to a standardized, bourgeois motherhood—particularized, in this case, to a French ideal. This linkup of maternity and medicine with cultural and national identity played a pivotal role in the assimilation of Jewish, immigrant, and otherwise "different" women throughout the Western industrialized world.[5] Medical men, and the women who supported their efforts through the sanitary movement, quickly realized that modern, medicalized maternity could also be a highly effective tool in the construction, classification, and maintenance of colonial power and hierarchies.[6]

The Western world, which amalgamated scientific medicine and the promise of inevitable, teleological progress into a "modern," messianic colonial project, had discovered a new route to the transformation of degenerate races, like Tunisian Jews, through the medicalization of maternity and motherhood. France, eager to spread this *mission civilisatrice* to her colonies, found an eager audience in the Jewish community of the Tunisian protectorate. Jewish elites in France and Tunisia had already advanced extensive efforts to modernize both the physical layout of Tunis (sanitary infrastructure, housing projects, etc.) and the perceived deficiencies of the Jewish body itself—a challenge undertaken by both the AIU and nascent Zionist movements. Within this group of colonial Jews, eager to demonstrate substantively their "Frenchness," the protectorate regime found a discrete population amenable to adopt the contemporary, scientific ideas surrounding modern childbirth and hygienic motherhood.

Reaching an acme in the late nineteenth and early twentieth centuries, French progressive reformers were increasingly preoccupied with the scientific connections between national strength and biological reproduction.[7] Amid fears of domestic decline, especially in the aftermath of "the defeat" in 1871 and the tenuous victory of World War I, French officials focused on redressing the precipitously declining French birthrate. Although metropolitan health officials by and large embraced hygienic interventions that promised some hope of national regeneration,[8] the boundaries between the included and the marginalized complicated the discourse surrounding fecundity and motherhood in the North African colonial context.[9] According to metropolitan officials, some segments of the colonial population were not ready or fit for modern scientific intervention. To wit, Muslim women in Tunisia were generally ignored or excluded from metropolitan efforts to export modernized maternity to the colonial setting. This lack of interest on the part of French officials, who considered Muslims as "unassimilable," was exacerbated by the indigenous, cultural norm of segregating Muslim women from both men and "nonbelievers."[10]

In contrast to the general apathy toward the Muslim population, French officials incorporated Tunisia's Jews into their drive toward medicalized maternity. The inclusion of Tunisian Jews in French colonial reproductive schemes was likely due to several interrelated factors. First, there was already an established metropolitan tradition of attempts to modernize and assimilate Jews into the national fabric of France.[11] The appeal to include Jews as part of the French nation dates back to Abbé Henri Grégoire's prerevolutionary essay, which advocated "the physical, moral, and political regeneration of the Jews."[12] A strong metropolitan lobby of Jews, best represented by the "founding fathers" of the AIU, transported this idea of Jewish acculturation and "rehabilitation" to the colonial environment.[13] Muslims, on the other hand, lacked an influential metropolitan presence that could lobby for the interests of its coreligionists. By the dawn of the twentieth century, the efforts to incorporate Jews into the national composition of France, domestically and in the colonies, focused more overtly on female reproduction and domesticity.

A second factor militating toward the inclusion of Tunisian Jews in the push for medicalized maternity was the French government's fervent desire to outpace the Italian population in the Tunisian protectorate. The 1910 census of the Tunisian protectorate showed that 105,000 Italian nationals grossly outnumbered the 35,000 French in Tunisia.[14] To augment the lagging French population, colonial officials gradually eased citizenship requirements to handpicked individuals between 1910 and 1923, almost exclusively Jewish men (and their prospective offspring).[15] To increase the number of Tunisian Jews fully acculturated to French normative values and ready to assume the responsibilities incumbent on French citizens, colonial officials and their allies realized that interventions in the Tunisian Jewish community must start early and concentrate on the intimate level of reproduction and domesticity. According to the dictates of science, only healthy, well-informed women under the watchful eyes of male physicians could produce vigorous offspring, and only properly trained mothers could raise these offspring as "French" children.

After World War I, the focus shifted from the medicalization of biological childbirth to the medicalization of social motherhood. According to this view, the social and cultural atmosphere of one's upbringing, coupled with the inculcation of proper hygienic practices, played a much larger role in cultivating Frenchmen than scrutiny over the biological process of birth. The initial indicators of acculturation—the acquisition of the basic markers of the larger society, such as language, dress, and the more amorphous category of "values"[16]—were learned primarily during childhood.

In the metropole French Jews meticulously cultivated their image as valuable and cooperative citizens within French society.[17] Similarly, in North Africa Jewish men played an instrumental role in helping the French navigate the "Arab" world.[18] French authorities, apparently oblivious to the economic, political, and social benefits derived by Jews from their role as mediators, instead characterized their Jewish collaborators as timid, subservient, and obliging.[19] In contradistinction to the purported obsequiousness of Tunisia's mild-mannered, Jewish men, French travelogues remarked on the disruptive vulgarity (and beauty) of Jewish women, who, unlike their Muslim sisters, circulated freely through the streets of Tunis.[20] The gaudiness and impropriety of these unacculturated women, who clung to "Arab" ways and failed to accept and practice French "good manners," shocked elite Jews and colonial officials.[21] The mastery of correct social behavior and proper etiquette offered by the French civilizing mission was part of an extensive skill set through which Tunisian Jewish women could prove not only their conquest over innate barbarism but also their ability to raise future generations of Frenchmen.[22] Jewish women in Tunisia, described as "noisy, curious, untidy, careless women," were subjected to a confusing array of contradictory messages.[23] For instance, although the French savagely decried their garishness and immodesty, Jewish community leaders criticized Jewish women who veiled themselves with "Arab-like" modesty and "suspected [veiled Jewish women] of engaging in intrigues or clandestine outings."[24]

Any possible intriguing aside, truculent "Arab" Jews in Tunisia presented much the same challenge to the process of quiescent acculturation as "traditional" eastern Jewish émigrés did in the metropole.[25] Upper-echelon Jews realized that their social and political status in both France and Tunisia was inextricably linked to the mores of Jews as a collective. Marginalized Jews who flouted French bourgeois behavioral norms reflected badly on those who fervently toed the line. Complicating the absorption of eastern Jews into the community of metropolitan French Jews was the fact that between 1872 and 1907 two-thirds of these immigrants were men.[26] This forced homosociality, which exacerbated the "queerness" of eastern Jewish culture in the eyes of metropolitan French Jews, placed added stress on the domestic acculturation process.[27] In contrast, French Jews and their allies viewed working-class Tunisian Jewish women as fertile targets for their reformative message and acculturation schemes. Jewish women carried the health and social hygienic ambitions of the French *mission civilisatrice* to places men alone could not reach—the domestic arena, child-rearing practices, and the reproductive sphere.

Women Spread the Gospel of Germs

In interwar Tunis (1919–39) roughly a fifth of the Jewish population belonged to the privileged class. These families lived in detached villas equipped with separate spaces for dining, sleeping, and congregating. Their spacious homes had modern furniture, Oriental carpets, and rich draperies, but also kitchens with electric refrigeration and private bathroom facilities. In many aspects, their domestic arrangements mirrored those of bourgeois households in the metropole. In contrast, the majority of the Jewish population of interwar Tunis—about 60 percent—belonged to a broadly defined middle class. For these families, space was at a premium. Extended family units shared one or two rooms in which all family members collectively dined, slept, and congregated. Sparse furnishings were passed from one generation to the next, and kitchen and bathroom facilities were shared with multiple neighbors. Parents and children usually shared a common bed. In many ways, for those at the middle and bottom of the socioeconomic ladder, life was a public spectacle and a collective struggle. Most lodgings faced a courtyard, where the children played, and doors to individual dwellings were rarely closed. Women prepared meals and did household chores while calling out to one another, exchanging recipes or domestic items. Women cooked, washed, and sewed on their doorsteps and commented freely on each neighbor's lot in life.[28]

Into this milieu of camaraderie and shared sacrifice, privileged Jewish women carried the French civilizing mission and its message of the hygienic household and modern child-rearing strategies. The sanitary movement of the late nineteenth century, together with the rise of public health movements in the early twentieth century, increased exponentially the role and responsibility of women in the domestic arena. Wealthy Jewish women in Tunis were the principle emissaries of the hygienic "good news," and they understood that only a carefully tailored message of modern French values could successfully penetrate the carefully guarded realm of Jewish motherhood. Women, who had always been in charge of the domestic sphere, now assumed the added responsibility of keeping the home—and the children—not just "clean," but free from "microbes."

Cleanliness, nutrition, and vigilant oversight were crucial to raising healthy offspring. These tasks, hitherto included within a subset of so-called motherly emotions, morphed into a set of behaviors and activities that were not innately or "naturally" known by good mothers.[29] Good mothers needed modern medico-scientific instruction to successfully raise healthy French citizens. The fact that the recipients of this new medical and scientific message did not have the financial resources to claim bourgeois status (and all its modern, time-reducing trappings) was irrelevant. Elite Jewish women argued that their lesser-privileged sisters could aspire to manners of status without possessing the means.[30] Cleanliness, modernity, and order were not the exclusive advantage of those who possessed the accouterments of wealth.

In 1952 a Scottish demographer noted that the extremely high birthrate among Muslim women in Tunisia was "a social and psychological question, with its roots reaching deep into the fundamental principles of Islam." Although Western medical ideas, such as birth control, had infiltrated Tunisian Jewish life, the demographer lamented, "Islam in North Africa has not witnessed the complete breakdown of its traditional family systems."[31] In spite of this demographer's assumption, the "traditional family system" of Jews in Tunisia had not broken down, but women were making the conscious choice to limit their family size. The birthrate among Jewish women fell from 45 per 1,000 before 1914 to just over 30 per 1,000 from 1934 to 1938.[32] It seems likely that a discussion of birth control practices became part of the "gospel" that women disseminated throughout their feminine networks and that elite as well as working-class women were receptive to its message.[33]

The endeavor to spread the "good news" of cleanliness, nutrition, proper child care, and birth control elevated the status of bourgeois women, and they struggled to build on their success and resist further male encroachments. A vivid example of this resistance to male authority can be seen in the statutory modifications of the Jewish Maternity Assistance (Mutualité Maternelle Israélite) plan. The plan, founded in 1905, provided monetary relief to indigent Jewish women in labor; gave access to doctors, midwives, and mohelim (circumcisers); furnished necessary clothing for the newborn; and when needed, assigned a wet nurse. The allocation of resources and decisions regarding the administration of services was assigned to a decision-making body of seven men, three of whom were required to be mohelim. This executive body was elected by a majority vote of members—membership was restricted to Jewish men who paid forty francs in yearly dues.[34]

Prominent women in the Tunis Jewish community derided the scheme and the overwhelming control that it allotted to male community members. They asserted that only women were qualified to advise on health matters that affected the lives of other women and their offspring. Women, whether indigent or privileged, should not be compelled to submit to male dominance over intimate, female space. In the face of women's widespread refusal to support the scheme, the plan's male members were forced back to the drawing board. In 1910 the statutory guidelines of the assistance plan were modified to include as participants in the plan's membership "any person who pays 20 centimes a month dues." Article 6 specified that "any person" was restricted to mean "only women." Furthermore, article 7 was amended to allow that "female participants, who have been members for more than one month, are granted the privilege to oversee cases with which they have a familiarity greater than that of the Société [male members]."[35] In other words, female "participants" had the clout to trump the opinion and judgment of male "members." In this instance, women maintained their long-standing control of the birthing room and attendant charitable schemes in spite of efforts by male physicians to supplant female authority.

A contemporary account of life in interwar Tunis noted that although patriarchal authority was the fundamental organizing principle of the Jewish family "in theory"; in fact, the mother's authority was "preponderant concerning upbringing and education."[36] Those tasked with acculturating wayward Tunisian Jewish women to French bourgeois values lamented that "[indigenous Jewish women] have no discernment and no knack for the little touches by which a good housewife succeeds in making her home attractive and comfortable. In addition, these women are apathetic; they are ignorant of the most elementary rules of polite conduct and personal hygiene. *They don't even know how to care for their children* [emphasis mine]."[37]

In regard to this most essential care—adequate food and nutrition—surveys conducted just before World War II revealed that 60 percent of Tunisians were malnourished, 40 percent severely so.[38] One-third of daily caloric intake was empty carbohydrates (mostly bread), and although Tunisia produced more than enough olive oil to supplement the fat intake of its citizens, it was far too dear to consume domestically. In spite of the evidence demonstrating the dearth of food, acculturated Jews insisted that "maternal apathy" caused the misery and malnutrition of Jewish children in Tunis.[39] "Their [Jewish mothers] treatment of children runs counter to all common sense; they regulate neither what, nor when their children eat. This is true to such a degree that the doctor at the dispensary [in Tunis] was obliged to pay for criers to make announcements so the mothers would know to feed their children every three hours."[40] In many ways, this quote speaks to the disconnection between the lives of those Jewish women at the apex of the economic hierarchy and those at the bottom and to the fundamental ways in which they misapprehended the hand-to-mouth existence of their less fortunate sisters. In all fairness, prosperous Jewish women did work tirelessly to disseminate the "gospel of germs" and healthful domesticity to the masses. Jewish charities, organized primarily by wealthy Jewish women, held numerous philanthropic events in Tunis. These balls, costume parties, and other gala events raised money to defray the cost associated with raising underprivileged Jewish children in the "proper" fashion and remolding the slatternly lifestyles of poor Jews. Although condescending in their own way, these Jewish charities purchased thousands of shoes and sweaters for needy children and provided hundreds of thousands of free meals to indigent children.[41]

However, elite Jews noted that there was a fine line between providing assistance to the responsible "deserving poor" and condoning the reckless lifestyle of the inveterately lazy. Noblesse oblige was neither without limits nor without conditions. Part of good morality implied playing by the rules, and colonial officials and elite Jews were vigilantly on guard against those who would abuse the system and try to profit from the largesse of others. To that end, the women "participants" of the Jewish Maternity Assistance plan requested a modification of the statutory guidelines in order to crack down on suspected freeloaders. The modified statutes of the plan provided foodstuffs for indigent mothers in lieu of monetary relief.[42] The direct provision of "milk, meat, eggs, etc." avoided any risk that needy women would spend cash assistance on frivolous or unnecessary items.

Colonial officials voiced similar concerns regarding abuse of the French *goutte de lait* (milk dispensary) in Makhtar, Tunisia (southwest of Tunis). The dispensary was supposed to provide "well-baby" services to the local population, as well as necessities like soap and milk. However, according to complaints received by the inspector of social hygiene, "the babies are not examined, nor weighed, and quite often are not even present. The names of those who receive services are listed in a registry, which has made it easy to ascertain that many of the recipients do not even have babies."[43] As an example of the degree of "waste," colonial officials noted, "in 1935, we have distributed over 1,754 containers of milk for 24 registered babies."[44]

Another common complaint leveled at indigenous women was that they perpetuated and exacerbated the deleterious effects of outdated and dangerous folk practices and superstitions. According to folkways, the seemingly benign act of complimenting the health or fine appearance of a child extended an invitation to jealous spirits or "evil eye" to harm the child.[45] French-trained health advocates noted, "You must be careful not to compliment the mother when you see a beautiful infant; when the least little thing goes wrong *as a result of her negligence or lack of hygiene*, she will accuse you of having put a curse on him!"[46] To ward off evil eye, there were various apotropaic talismans and folk practices that could assist anxious mothers, such as a pair of scissors and a Hebrew book placed under the child's pillow or a "hand of Miriam" ("hand of Fatima" for Muslims) posted at the entry to the child's room.

An additional folk practice that irritated the French and their acculturated colleagues was that Jewish women abstained from postpartum breast-feeding for several days and relied instead on the assistance of wet nurses. Acculturated Jews lamented, "As a result of [unacculturated Jewish women's] ignorance [in other words, by not breast-feeding], the baby suffers from horrible colic and diarrhea, to which he is lost more often than not."[47] To combat this dangerous practice, the female "participants" of the Jewish Maternity Assistance plan intervened once again and insisted that male members had been far too liberal regarding the allowance of wet nurses to indigent mothers. As a result, the modified statutes of 1910 limited the provision of wet nurses to indigent parturient mothers when "absolutely necessary" and "only . . . as resources permit."[48]

Physicians, adherents of the AIU, and their public health allies in the protectorate regime complained that unacculturated Jewish women failed to safely manage domestic responsibilities and that negligence and indifference exacerbated infant morbidity and mortality. According to these claims, Jewish babies that survived infancy faced the prospect of a dangerous childhood during which they would not be watched or tended by their mothers.[49] However, in spite of all of the claims of ignorance and neglect leveled at underprivileged Jewish women, in truth, the mass of the evidence shows that these mothers were quite attentive, if not doting. Jewish mothers, regardless of social standing, were also quick to adopt any form of "modernity" that demonstrated a benefit or advantage for their children.

On October 12, 1912, the director of the AIU school came upon what he perceived to be a riot in front of his school. "We are besieged!" he wrote. "The assailants' intentions cannot be mistaken: they would take our building by storm. The police must be summoned without delay." Three policemen arrived to hold the throngs at bay, but the mob breached the interior of the school.

> The floodgates burst open and the wave of humanity, all the stronger for having been so long contained, pours into every corner of the school, rises up stairs, inundates corridors, and overruns classrooms. The ill-fated headmistress and her heroic assistant are at the mercy of the crowd. They lose their footing and are tossed about in the storm until they suddenly feel the grope of strong hands and find themselves, as if by miracle, shut into the head office. They have bumps and bruises; their poor feet are beaten to a pulp. Yet, feeling this is a small price to pay for having escaped the threatening crowd, they breathe not a word of complaint. A passerby, intrigued by this mad scramble, asks what is the reason for it. Someone says in reply, Today is the day registration forms are distributed at the Alliance school for girls.[50]

This example, which refers directly to indigent women in the Jewish ghetto, demonstrates that these mothers were hardly indifferent or apathetic in regard to their children. One contemporary noted in 1922, "[Jewish] girls go to school just as boys, but in separate establishments. In Tunis, the schools of the Alliance Israélite have around 4,200 boys and 3,800 girls."[51] While at school, children were under the watchful eye of the alliance instructors, who closely examined each child's cleanliness. The blue uniform and beret were mandatory, and "each morning the teachers lined up the students for physical examination, insisting on correct posture and good personal hygiene. They verified, among other things, the cleanliness of the head, the ears, and the nails. Teachers did not hesitate to pull a student out by the ear if he or she had dirty ears, and the same thing went for shoes, which had to be brushed and polished."[52] Outside school mothers remained on guard for the slightest injury to their offspring. Some mothers relied on folkways and herbal medicine to care for injuries; they applied a plaster of crushed, salted onions to wounds. Children complained that the malodorous poultice, although effective, also quarantined them from their playmates. The clumsiest children were often spotted with the red marks of Mercurochrome, which every mother had in her medicine cabinet.[53] As these examples show, each woman, whether teacher or mother, French or Tunisian, rich or poor, played a role in the drama of colonialism and in the dissemination of the gospel of germs. These women should not be relegated to a monolithic, isolated entity that "belonged to" either the colonizer or the colonized. At "all stages of the imperial enterprise the experiences of these two groups of women were intertwined," and we should consider their stories as fragments of a single, cohesive, albeit complicated historical narrative.[54]

Men Saving (Jewish) Babies

Between 1909 and 1928, 117 per 1,000 babies born to French women in Tunisia did not survive the first year of life. The mortality rate increased to 175 per 1,000 for Jews and to 236 per 1,000 for Muslims.[55] The medical establishment opined that the only way to decrease high mortality rates of parturient mothers and newborns—to bring the vital statistics of Jews closer to French—was through a modern, scientific approach to childbirth and motherhood. Male physicians and sanitarians claimed that their modern approach—displacement of traditional birth attendants by obstetricians, the surveillance of pregnancy by medical professionals, a shift in the location of childbirth from the home to institutional settings, and an increase in the number of obstetrical interventions—could save mothers and babies.[56] Colonial officials together with elite Jews in Paris and Tunis (men) worked to bring these gifts of medicalized maternity and motherhood to Tunis's less fortunate Jews. In many ways, the exclusion of Muslim women only increased the social prestige of medicalized motherhood among Jewish women who sought to define themselves as separate from "Arab" practices and amenable to French normative cultural behaviors.[57] Accepting medicalized motherhood with all its trappings became a desirable symbol of French acculturation among Jewish women in Tunis—one that denoted upward social mobility, rational thought, and progress.

But male physicians wondered (aloud) if women could adequately manage oversight of a biological process so governed by the complex laws of science. Although the medico-scientific patriarchy recognized that women were more adept at nurturing and administering "kindness," women, according to these same savants, were not socially or even mentally equipped to cope with, let alone understand, the more complex scientific and medical aspects of their own bodies. Permitting "respectable" women access to delicate information in relation to their own physiology was a prospect that displeased the male medical establishment. The most effective method of monitoring and controlling childbirth was to move the entire process into the male-centered, medical environment of the hospital maternity ward.

In spite of their bold plans, the French-led medical establishment and its advocates found that relocating childbirth to the maternity ward would prove far more difficult than anticipated. The primary obstacle was a lack of facilities staffed by French-trained male physicians able to oversee childbirth in full compliance with the 1888 legislation requiring governmental oversight of all medical practice in Tunisia.[58] When the Jewish Hospital (*l'hôpital israélite*) in Tunis opened its doors in the Place Halfaouine in 1895, it contained a scant total of forty beds staffed by five physicians who addressed only the direst needs of the community. In conformity with the colonial push to provide modern childbirth to Tunisian Jewish women, the Jewish Hospital established a maternity ward in 1910. However, the hospital, which was only adequately equipped to treat acute emergencies, could not maintain an open-door policy for parturient women. To avoid swamping the limited resources of the hospital and its staff, the community grappled with effective strategies to ration medical care.

The Jewish community decided that the most utilitarian option was to allocate its limited maternity space to repentant "fallen" or "abandoned" women outside the traditional support structure provided by female midwives and relatives. Hence, the statutes of the hospital, drawn up by the all-male Tunis Jewish Community Council (Conseil de la communauté israélite de Tunis), reserved the maternity ward for the use of Jewish women who could prove their "worthiness and indigence" *and* obtain authorization, in the form of an "admission coupon," from the aforementioned all-male council.[59] In spite of the goal to elevate the allure of hospital birth among Jewish women, the decisions of the Tunis Jewish Community Council had the contradictory effect. As a result of the draconian and humiliating admission requirements, only the most forlorn women availed themselves, or were forced to submit to, the ignominy of hospital childbirth.

The disparity between lofty aspirations and meager resources that stymied attempts to implement hospital childbirth at the community level was mirrored at the "national" colonial level. In spite of the desire by physicians and colonial authorities to move French women (and those Jewish women who were amenable to acculturation) into the male-supervised world of the hospital maternity ward, the lack of adequate infrastructure and staffing made this impossible. For all of their talk of medicalizing maternity through hospital-centered childbirth, male physicians and the protectorate regime allotted little time and few resources to realize the goal. Between 1910 and 1930, maternity wards in Tunis opened no additional bed space. In 1930 the French hospital in Tunis (*l'hôpital civil français*) opened a small maternity ward for the express use of indigent French women. Once again, rationing hospital childbirth to serve only the most socially marginalized women engendered the undesired effect of reducing the allure and prestige of hospital births among women who sought modern bourgeois status. In 1931 only 3.65 percent of European and Jewish women in Tunisia gave birth in a hospital.[60] As a result, until more resources could be allotted to building and staffing adequate numbers of maternity wards, the focus of modernizing maternity would have to rely on the control and inspection of home births.[61]

While the aspiration of the French medical establishment and its advocates to relocate childbirth to the hospital setting was materially unrealizable, the goal to oversee pregnancy and birth within the home was even more problematic. In the early twentieth century, unlicensed female elders (*matrones*) still supervised the majority of births in Tunisia without the presence of a male physician.[62] To track (and intimidate) these unlicensed practitioners who purportedly threatened the lives of parturient women, Dr. Reynal, chief of the Tunis Office of Municipal Hygiene in Tunis, mandated in 1930 the registration of every birth along with the name(s) of the elder, midwife, or physician who attended the birth.[63] However, it was not only the scientifically untrained *matrones* that harmed babies and parturient mothers. According to male physicians trained in the science of obstetrics, even *licensed* midwives (*sage-femmes*) had failed to master lifesaving scientific knowledge. Midwives, who learned by traditional empiricism, passed their knowledge to their daughters, who, according to a contemporary male physician, "inherit from their mothers' scientific incompetence and total negligence regarding hygienic practices."[64] Especially worrisome, according to physicians, was the unsupervised administration of the drug oxytocin to speed uterine contractions and precipitate delivery. Midwives, regardless of training, were not a substitute for the skill and knowledge of male physicians, especially gynecologists and obstetricians.

But regardless of their purported skills, the number of licensed physicians in Tunisia was very low. In 1892 there were 106 physicians permitted to practice in Tunisia, forty-seven of whom held European diplomas.[65] By 1933 the number of practicing physicians in Tunisia had risen to 364.[66] However, for a population of more than two million, the ratio of physicians to patients (about 1:5,500) was de minimis.[67] Yet in spite of their relative rarity, physicians led a precarious economic existence. Contemporary reports allege that "less than half" of all patients were "desirable," in other words, able to pay for medical care.[68] Taking this factor into account, the push by physicians to enter the birthing room takes on new significance. Physicians did not want indiscriminate access to birthing rooms per se; they desired access to parturient mothers who were willing to be acculturated to French normative values and, most important, able to pay a fee. Despite the small number of licensed physicians in Tunisia, internal market pressures forced them to fight for a marginal slice within a limited pie chart of paying patients. Moreover, there was a growing uneasiness regarding the advent of centralized, government-led health-care initiatives. In short, physicians were struggling to solidify their fragile professional authority and to protect their economic self-interest from the specter of socialized medicine.[69]

In 1905 two physicians working for the Tunisian health service (i.e., civil servants, not private practitioners) published a proposal in the *Revue tunisienne* calling for the establishment of a medical social safety net that would extend the care of licensed physicians to all Tunisians. According to their plan, a modest tax of three or four francs levied on indigenous Tunisians could support a nationwide medical staff. However, physicians refused, en masse, to submit to a scheme that not only mandated a fixed civil servant's salary but also implied possible relocation to a Saharan outpost. The plan was never implemented.[70] As in mainland France, physicians in Tunisia warned that direct government control of any aspect of the medical marketplace created a slippery slope toward socialized medicine and would be the death knell for private practice.

Physicians also bemoaned the high number of unlicensed women who "practiced medicine" in Tunisia. They feared that the presence of cheaper medical alternatives (*matrones* and *sage-femmes*) usurped their economic power and distorted the medical marketplace. To avert the dilution of their medical monopoly, physicians lobbied the protectorate regime to limit the number of practitioners licensed to assist childbirth. The number of trained midwives in Tunis was already low—in 1920 there were only thirty-seven. To assuage the fears of physicians, the Bureau of Hygiene in Tunis assumed control of midwifery training in 1928, and in 1935 the municipality licensed and hired seven midwives. To avoid economic competition, these new municipal midwives were barred from assisting women whom the city judged "able to pay." In 1931 the municipal midwives assisted just 42 of the 7,459 live births in Tunis.[71]

It seems fair to assume that doctors wanted to inhibit parturient women from establishing a rapport with female medical practitioners (licensed or unlicensed) on whom they might call in cases of further medical emergencies. Physicians, for their part, aspired to be the only "legitimate" source of medical assistance. Despite their stated goal to modernize and medicalize childbirth in Tunis, the evidence indicates that French-trained physicians were also very cognizant of their precarious economic condition. They realized that any provider—male or female, licensed or unlicensed—who assisted childbirth established an important bond with the parturient mother and her newborn infant. Medical practice, then as today, was an intensely personal relationship, and the medical provider who treated the mother usually treated the entire family. The birthing room served in many ways as a point of access to the intimate domestic sphere and established a toehold from which an industrious medical practitioner could expand his or her practice. Individual physicians and the regime recognized the potential economic importance of these relationships and jealously fought to keep them within their exclusive domain.

Preserving a physician's economic prerogative from internal threats (women) was par for the course, but one striking example from Tunis in 1933 illustrates just how far the protectorate regime was willing to go to protect economic turf from external male threats. From the earliest days of the protectorate, the French administration had allowed any physician with a diploma, regardless of nationality, to practice medicine in Tunisia. However, as previously mentioned, by the interwar years, the protectorate regime suddenly alleged (in the face of overwhelming counterevidence) a surfeit of physicians. In 1933 Resident General Marcel Peyrouton received nearly fifty requests from German-Jewish physicians seeking permission to flee Nazi Germany and establish medical practice in Tunisia. According to Peyrouton, the voice of the Tunisian regime, the "medical proletariat" was already flooded with "Jews who could not support themselves." In spite of repeated pleas by Pierre-Etienne Flandin, the French minister of foreign affairs, Peyrouton refused to grant asylum to the doctors. In a terse response to Flandin's request, Peyrouton responded that he would like Minister Flandin "to explain to him what his attitude *should be* towards these German-Jews wishing to practice medicine in Tunis."[72] Peyrouton also ordered the summary deportation of all physicians who moved directly to Tunisia without obtaining prior permission. In March 1937 the protectorate barred the practice of all foreign doctors owing to the "oversupply of physicians in Tunisia."[73]

It is difficult to pinpoint the motivations of various actors in the French colonial regime in blocking the entry of the Jewish doctors. In light of contemporary attitudes toward Jews, racial animus cannot be discounted.[74] But it is also worth noting that by the early 1930s, the Great Depression had extended its tentacles to the periphery of the French Empire, and professional unions (and medical lobbying groups) were becoming increasingly jealous and protective of their economic prerogatives. Moreover, in 1932 the French population of Tunisia had finally surpassed that of the Italians; hence, the French government no longer needed additional Jewish naturalizations to achieve demographic domination.

By the end of the nineteenth century, Western medicine had supplanted "traditional medicine" in Tunisia, and French-trained male physicians of all faiths sought to represent themselves as a united science-based profession.[75] But under the veneer of unity, male physicians in Tunis were engaged in a desperate struggle to grab their share of the limited paying patient-base. Supervision of childbirth allowed "outside" men to establish an economic foothold within the "inside" sphere of patient-rich female domestic networks. Men enacted restrictive legislation and reduced training opportunities in order to limit female midwifery. Male physicians and the protectorate regime also worked to resist the "socialization" of childbirth and to bar "foreign" physicians from practicing medicine in Tunisia. In spite of their rhetoric advocating the extension of the salutary benefits of "modern" childbirth to all Tunisian women, physicians were, in fact, overtly jockeying to expand and safeguard their economic terrain. In light of the limited role played by male physicians in childbirth and child rearing, historians must consider that "women's work" undertaken by Jewish female networks significantly reduced—perhaps more than male physicians—the morbidity and mortality rates of parturient Jewish women and children in Tunis during the interwar era.

Statistical data collected between 1911 and 1926 showed that the Jewish infant mortality rate in Tunisia closely mirrored that of the French. Each peaked in 1916 and fell every subsequent year until 1926. Jewish infant mortality was 62.3 per 1,000 births in 1916 and by 1926 had fallen to 48.3 per 1,000. Over the same period, Muslim infant mortality steadily increased, reaching the tragic level of 82.0 per 1,000 births by 1926.[76] Between 1919 and 1946, infant mortality in the Jewish community in Tunis dropped by 23 percent. Over this same period, the rate for Muslim children only fell by 5 percent.[77]

Although decreased Jewish infant morbidity and mortality during the protectorate era has been largely credited to the medical interventions of French men and the Jewish men they trained, this narrow view of historical events ignores the important contributions of Jewish women. Throughout this period, women retained firm control of both childbirth and the care of children, and in spite of scarce resources, they managed to cobble together a healthy existence for their families. The historical master narrative regarding Jewish life in Tunisia has failed to acknowledge the important debt owed to increased female scholarization, the vulgarization of the gospel of germs among the women of the broad Jewish middle class and their more poverty-stricken sisters, and the vast networks of women's charitable endeavors for the drastic decline in mortality rates of Jewish children after World War I. This account adds a "Judeo-colonial" example to the scholarship on women's counter-narratives to the assumed superiority of male-dominated science and medicine and the myriad ways in which women asserted modernity on their own terms.[78] While it is true that many Jewish women (and men) were hostile toward Western medical practices that eroded preexisting indigenous cultural and religious traditions, especially in the early years of the protectorate era, increased good health and lower infant mortality dampened opposition. It was difficult to argue against demonstrable results. This chapter reflects the difficulty expressed by many Jews—Tunisian and French, male and female—in trying to square the repressive and coercive messages of regeneration and assimilation with the apparent salubrious ramifications of colonial science and medicine. The increased availability of hospital childbirth, combined with better knowledge of obstetrics, prenatal care, and infant nutrition, became incorporated into the social fabric of what constituted common female expertise and know-how. Scientific authority, even when subconsciously acquired or absorbed through osmosis, was nonetheless a powerful component in convincing parturient mothers to join the quest toward regeneration—on their own terms.

Conclusion

A Brief Reflection on Identity

But I have no sense of humor and not enough courage to be cynical.

—ALBERT MEMMI, *The Colonizer and the Colonized*

On a warm and sunny spring day in March 2009, I sat in the Café El M'rabet on rue Souk Trok in the Tunis medina drinking strong coffee and fiddling with my digital camera, the more advanced features of which still elude me. At the table next to me, an elderly couple sipped their *thés aux pignons* and examined me in the inscrutable but smiling Tunisian way. Finally, the gentleman asked me what I was in the area to photograph. I explained to them that I had been taking photos of the housing complexes on the rue Dr. Cassar in the northern medina. At this point, the lady chimed in and volunteered that this area of Tunis was once a vibrant Jewish neighborhood but that the Jews had all gone years ago. She asked if I would like to know more about the Jews of Tunis, and I admitted that it was in fact my purpose for being in Tunisia. With a furtive glance at the tables next to us, she suggested that we meet outside to talk, as it was not safe to discuss such things in a public place. Of course, this was just before the revolution that toppled the repressive Ben Ali regime, and such fear was not uncommon, especially when speaking to a Westerner like myself.

Outside in the sun, we sat on the stoop of a neighboring building and chatted. I wondered aloud how she knew so much about the hara and the former Jewish community. Her partner leaned forward and whispered, "She's an Israélite. She was there." With his prompting, she reminisced about the three Jewish housing blocs built on rue Dr. Cassar and informed me quite without rancor that they were now "entirely Muslim." The area across the street, which was now surrounded by fencing and topped with concertina wire, had once housed a Jewish elementary school and one of the oldest synagogues in the Maghrib. The school and the synagogue had been destroyed in the 1960s to make way for a mosque and soccer field. Although it was impossible to see over the fences, I could hear children playing on the field. This elderly lady, whose name was never offered, recounted the disappearance of her community with surprising equanimity, recalling the dramatic events of the late 1960s and early 1970s that emptied Tunisia of all but a few remaining Jews. When I asked her why she stayed, she answered, as if surprised by the question, that she was Tunisian, so where else could she live?

When considered as a whole, the distinct accounts in this book have presented a brief narrative or snapshot of Jewish life in Tunisia under the French protectorate and the importance of regeneration to the construction of identity—the meanings embedded in modern space, the social and cultural grace of the French, the muscular pride of the Zionist, or the rising voices of contemporary women. By refracting detailed accounts of local stories through the lens of broader historical events and medico-scientific theories, we have examined the obscured exchanges and hidden structures of these new political, cultural, and social realities. Examining the quest for regeneration in the Tunisian Jewish community provides important connections between the opaque racialized theories of the late nineteenth century and the palpable brutality of early twentieth-century colonial interventions.

Regeneration, initiated in the Jewish community as a eugenic crusade supported by leading medical and scientific experts, evolved into a broader movement led by public health workers, hygienists, concerned citizens, and city planners equally eager to promote the health and well-being of their community. But again, I reiterate that regeneration was not a catalyst to inevitable modernization; it was a medically justified, scientifically based theory that shaped political, social, and cultural ideologies in unexpected and often counterintuitive ways. In spite of the power of scientific and medical authority, the responses and reactions to regeneration were as diverse as they were unforeseeable. The Tunisian Jewish community formed its own interpretations, manifestations, and expressions of modern identity and regeneration, which in many ways differed from, and even challenged, French beliefs. Extending the French discourses of acculturation, modernization, and regeneration to Jews in the Tunisian protectorate demonstrates that cultural group-identity and expression—what it meant to be a Jew, French, native, or metropolitan—was a contentious, ever-changing, and elaborate dance.

NOTES

1. Situating Regeneration

1. Degeneration was portrayed as a plague of the upper classes in Zola's *Pot-bouille* (1882), in J.-K. Huysmann's novel *A Rebours* (1884), and through Proust's iconic figure of moral decrepitude, the Baron de Charlus in *A la recherche du temps perdu* (1913–27). Emile Zola's Rougon-Macquart series also recounted degeneration in the lower or working classes: *L'Assomoir* (1877), *Nana* (1880), and *La bête humaine* (1890). However, race was not considered except as concerned the degeneration of the "French race."
2. Cooper and Stoler, *Tensions of Empire*; Clancy-Smith and Gouda, *Domesticating the Empire*; Stoler, *Carnal Knowledge and Imperial Power.*
3. Blumenbach et al., *On the Natural Varieties of Mankind*; Buffon, *Natural History*, vol. 4.
4. Lowney, *Vanished World*; Menocal, *Ornament of the World*; Lyons, *House of Wisdom*; Dodds, *Arts of Intimacy.*
5. Grégoire, *Essai sur la régénération.*
6. For a broad discussion of Abbé Grégoire's ideas, see Sepinwall, *Abbé Grégoire.*
7. Grégoire, *Motion en faveur des Juifs*, 27.
8. The ongoing effort of the French state to "normalize" relations with French Jews during the nineteenth century has been detailed in many works, including Graetz, *Jews in Nineteenth Century France*; Hyman, *Emancipation of the Jews of Alsace*; Benbassa, *Histoire des Juifs de France*; D. Cohen, *Promotion des Juifs en France*; Albert, "Israelite and Jew."
9. For works on the reach and influence of the AIU, see Rodrigue, *French Jews, Turkish Jews*; Rodrigue, *Images of Sephardi*; Laskier, *Alliance Israélite Universelle*; Chouraqui, *L'Alliance Israélite universelle*; Silberman, "Investigation of the Schools."
10. The Maghrib as a "border zone" of constructed identities has been examined in such works as Lorcin, *Imperial Identities*; Lorcin, *Kabyles, Arabs, Français*; Davis, *Resurrecting the Granary of Rome*; Rollman, "Some Reflections on Recent Trends"; Clancy-Smith, *North Africa, Islam and the Mediterranean World.*

11. Similar questions are considered in the Moroccan context: Schroeter and Chetrit, "Emancipation and Its Discontents"; Schroeter, "Shifting Boundaries of Moroccan Jewish Identities."
12. For an interesting microhistorical account of Algerian identity, see Bahloul, *Architecture of Memory*.
13. The sixth century BCE presence of Jews in Tunisia is mentioned not as a historical fact but as a commonly held "traditional" belief in Saadoun, "Tunisia," 445.
14. Sand, *Invention of the Jewish People*, 166–72, 199–209.
15. Stillman, *Jews of Arab Lands*, 44–45.
16. Stillman, *Jews of Arab Lands*, 77.
17. I use the term "port Jews" as defined by Lehmann, "Livornese 'Port Jew.'" For Sorkin's classic definition of a "port Jew," see Sorkin, "Port Jew." For Dubin's more expanded definition, see Dubin, *Port Jews of Habsburg Trieste*; Dubin, "Researching Port Jews and Port Jewries." Other terms have been proposed, such as "port-merchant" (see Catalan, *Ambivalence of a Port-City*) and "people of the diaspora" (see Monaco, "Port Jews or a People of the Diaspora?").
18. In addition to Italian Jews, many Italian (and Maltese) Christians settled in Tunisia as well. See Choate, "Identity Politics and Political Perception"; Clancy-Smith, "Gender in the City"; Sebag, *Tunis*; Del Piano, *La penetrazione italiana in Tunisia*; Ganiage, *Les origines du Protectorat français en Tunisie*.
19. Lehmann, "Livornese 'Port Jew,'" 70–71.
20. D. Cohen, *Le Parler Arabe des Juifs de Tunis*; Modena, "Spoken Languages of the Jews of Italy," 308.
21. Benjamin Hary, "Judeo-Arabic," Jewish Language Research Website, accessed October 27, 2011, www.jewish-languages.org/judeo-arabic.html.
22. Sebag, *Histoire des Juifs de Tunisie*, 261–62.
23. Sebag, *Histoire des Juifs de Tunisie*; Taïeb, "Grana (Livornese)."
24. Although ancestrally related to the rest of the Twansa community, Jews on the island of Jerba have long been (and still are) socially and culturally distinct from the "Tunisian" Jewish community. This proud but very insular community has its own unique history and identity that have been ably covered by Udovitch and Valensi, *Last Arab Jews*.
25. Schroeter, "Shifting Boundaries of Moroccan Jewish Identities," 147.
26. Lehmann, "Livornese 'Port Jew,'" 55, quoting Sorkin, "Port Jews," 88–89.
27. Lehmann, "Livornese 'Port Jew,'" 71.
28. Darwin, *De l'origine des espèces*.

29. Francis Galton did not coin the term "eugenics" until 1883, but its tenets were already well understood and being applied.
30. Efron, *Defenders of the Race*; Hart, *Healthy Jew*.
31. For an excellent explication of this French exceptionalism, see Schneider, *Quality and Quantity*.
32. Shepard, *Invention of Decolonization*, 13. Shepard notes the inherent tension between "scientific racism" and French universalism.
33. Schneider, *Quality and Quantity*, 9; Schneider, "Toward the Improvement of the Human Race"; Buican, "Sur le développement de la génétique classique en France," 240–41.
34. Schneider, "Toward the Improvement of the Human Race," 271; Conry, *L'Introduction du darwinisme en France au xixe siècle*.
35. Abi-Mershed, *Apostles of Modernity*.
36. For more on colonial prejudice and the construction of the "Orient," see Said, *Orientalism*; Arnold, *Colonizing the Body*; Bhabha, *Location of Culture*; Dirks, *Castes of Mind*. For such works with explicit reference to the Maghrib, see Benjamin, *Orientalist Aesthetics*; Kabbani, *Imperial Fictions*; Lowe, *Critical Terrains*.
37. Schechter, *Obstinate Hebrews*; Graetz, *Jews in Nineteenth Century France*; Berkovitz, *Shaping of Jewish Identity*; Albert, *Modernization of French Jewry*.
38. Rodrigue, *French Jews, Turkish Jews*; Rodrigue, *Images of Sephardi*; Laskier, *Alliance Israélite Universelle*; Chouraqui, *L'Alliance Israélite universelle*.
39. Latour, *We Have Never Been Modern*.
40. Said, *Orientalism*.
41. Bhabha, "Unsatisfied"; Bhabha, "Unpacking My Library," 210.
42. Dube and Banerjee-Dube, *Unbecoming Modern*, 4.
43. Gikandi, "Picasso, Africa, and the Schemata of Difference," 457.
44. Pratt, "Arts of the Contact Zone," 33–40; Pratt, *Imperial Eyes*. Historians and anthropologists have adopted and extended the meanings of Pratt's descriptions of language acquisition in the "contact zone" to include many culturally acquired behaviors in colonial space. Bhabha, *Location of Culture*, 55.
45. For a more in-depth discussion of the philosophical and Hegelian roots of colonial hybridity, see Nafafe, "Europe in Africa and Africa in Europe," 54.
46. This point has been ably demonstrated by such authors as Keller, *Colonial Madness*; and Tilley, *Africa as a Living Laboratory*.
47. Dube and Banerjee-Dube, *Unbecoming Modern*, 4.
48. Arnold, *Colonizing the Body*; Benjamin, *Orientalist Aesthetics*; Bhabha, *Location of Culture*; Dirks, *Castes of Mind*; Kabbani, *Imperial Fictions*; Keller, *Colonial Madness*;

Prakash, *Another Reason*; Said, *Orientalism*; Said, *Culture and Imperialism*; Spivak, *Critique of Postcolonial Reason*; Tilley, *Africa as a Living Laboratory*.

49. Conklin, *In the Museum of Man*; Osborne, *Emergence of Tropical Medicine in France*; Rabinow, *French Modern*; Conklin, *Mission to Civilize*; Wright, *Politics of Design in French Colonial Urbanism*; Wright, "Tradition in the Service of Modernity."
50. Conklin, *Mission to Civilize*, 5.
51. Adams and Reed, "Culture in the Transitions," 248–49.
52. Schreier, *Arabs of the Jewish Faith*; Abi-Mershed, *Apostles of Modernity*; Fischer-Tiné and Mann, *Colonialism as Civilizing Mission*; Betts, *Assimilation and Association*; Conklin, *Mission to Civilize*.
53. Wilder, *French Imperial Nation-State*, 6–8.
54. Wilder, *French Imperial Nation-State*, 6–8; Celestin and DalMolin, *France from 1851 to the Present*, 5. The critiques of Wilder, Celestin, and DalMolin are well taken; historians must be mindful of archival biases and the tensions that exist between French republican universalism and modernity. See also Steedman, *Dust*; Stoler, *Along the Archival Grain*; Stoler, *Imperial Debris*.
55. Todd Shepard provides an excellent analysis of the lasting trauma of French colonialism in Algeria and the painful legacy of decolonization, in *Invention of Decolonization*, 229–47.
56. Daughton, *Empire Divided*, 13, 16. Daughton notes that much policy in French colonial space was not ideologically motivated but rather more "practical" in its inspiration and application. Expanding on this point, I contend that many claim that there is a distinction between ideologically driven policies and those spawned by the imperatives of scientific authority, which rely on a direct appeal to logical and empirical references. See Canestrari, "Relationship between Ideology and Science."
57. Kuhn, *Structure of Scientific Revolutions*. Kuhn argues that our understanding of science (and medicine) cannot be established or rely solely on "objective facts." Subjective perspectives play an important role in forming our Weltanschauung. For a broad theoretical discussion of the power of experts in society, see Haskell, *Authority of Experts*.
58. L. Hunt, "French History in the Last Twenty Years."
59. Barnes, *Great Stink of Paris*, 6, citing Revel, *Jeux d'échelles*, 28.
60. Barnes, *Great Stink of Paris*, 6, citing Revel, *Jeux d'échelles*, 28; Chartier, *Cultural History*.
61. Adams and Reed, "Culture in the Transitions," 250.
62. Catro-Gómez, "Social Sciences, Epistemic Violence,'" 215–16; Dube, *Stiches on Time*, 7.

63. Dube and Banerjee-Dube, *Unbecoming Modern*, 217–18, quoting Blaut, *Colonizer's Model of the World*, 187.
64. Daughton, *Empire Divided*; White and Daughton, *In God's Empire*.
65. Cooper, *Colonialism in Question*, 67.

2. Regenerating Space

1. For a summation of the events leading up to Charles X's ignominious fall from power, see Pilbeam, "Growth of Liberalism." For a complete history of the French conquest of Algeria, see Sessions, *By Sword and Plow*; Abi-Mershed, *Apostles of Modernity*; Brower, *Desert Named Peace*.
2. The Crémieux Decree, signed October 24, 1870, naturalized en masse the Jews living in the three French departments of Algeria. The decree did not extend to Jews in southern Algeria or to any Muslims. "The Israelites native to the departments of Algeria are declared French citizens; consequently, their real status and their personal status shall be, dating from the promulgation of the present decree, regulated by French law, with all rights acquired until this day inviolable." The Crémieux Decree, Decree of October 24, 1870, VIII, 136, accessed October 27, 2011, www.akadem.org/photos/contextuels/4171_2_DecretCremieux.pdf.
3. I use the term "Tunisian Jews" in reference to "*tunisois* Jews," meaning Jews of Tunis. This book is for the most part limited to an examination of the Tunis Jewish community. Other Jewish communities in Tunisia, such as the Jerban community, have their own particularities and lie beyond the scope of my analysis. For more on Jerban Jewry, see Udovitch and Valensi, *Last Arab Jews*.
4. Perkins, *History of Modern Tunisia*, 40.
5. Aldrich, *Greater France*, 30.
6. For a description of the status of Italians in Tunisia, see Lewis, *Divided Rule*, 127.
7. As noted elsewhere in this book, many areas of the Tunis metropolitan area were perceived as Jewish or "non-Arab" space (like the hara or La Goulette) even though these areas were zones of mixed religious and ethnic affiliation.
8. In the farthest reaches of the Saharan desert in southern Tunisia, the military remained in control, ostensibly to guard the border with Tripolitania (Libya), which was seized by Italy in 1911 from the Ottoman Empire.
9. Perkins, *History of Modern Tunisia*, 87.
10. The precise numbers of French and indigenous members altered slightly over the years. These numbers represent those established in 1928. Braunschvig, "Tunisia."
11. Perkins, *History of Modern Tunisia*, 82.

12. Perkins, *History of Modern Tunisia*, 43. There were some exceptions to this rule: extreme southern Tunisia (the Saharan Desert) remained under military control to "protect" the border with Tripolitania.
13. Gallagher, *Medicine and Power*, 41–42.
14. Gallagher, *Medicine and Power*, 92–93.
15. Archives de l'Institut Pasteur (AIP) FR BUR, dossier of Etienne Burnet.
16. The use of public health administrative powers to effect sweeping changes in Tunisia is outlined in Gaumer, *L'organisation*.
17. Cohen and Johnson, *Filth*, xxvii.
18. The increased regulation of the sanitary infrastructure of Tunis and La Goulette can be seen in Gaumer's *L'organisation* and in the codification of such practices in chapter 5 of the Commune de la Goulette's "Règlement de la voirie" of 1929.
19. Schlör, *Nights in the Big City*; Maxwell, *Mysteries of Paris and London*; Marcus, *Apartment Stories*.
20. Marcotte, *L'art de bâtir*, 392.
21. Dedet, *Les Institute Pasteur d'outre-mer*, 70; Gallagher, *Medicine and Power*, 7.
22. Sebag, *Tunis*, 354.
23. Commune de la Goulette, "Règlement de la voirie," Chapter V, Section 3, Article 85, 1929.
24. Commune de la Goulette, "Règlement de la voirie," Chapter V, Section 3, Article 84, 1929.
25. Commune de la Goulette, "Règlement sanitaire," Title II, Article 46, 1929.
26. Commune de la Goulette, "Règlement sanitaire," Title II, Articles 49 and 50, 1929.
27. Commune de la Goulette, "Règlement sanitaire," Title II, Article 23, 1929.
28. Gaumer, *L'organisation*, 172.
29. I pluralize "*funduq*" and "*wakāla*" by adding an "s" as these transliterations are commonly used in English and French. The correct Arabic plurals would be *funādiq* and *wakālāt*.
30. Raymond, *Grandes villes arabes à l'époque ottomane*.
31. The nineteenth-century transition from miasmatic theory to germ theory of disease causation—sparking widespread intellectual uncertainty, scientific debates, and public confusion and conflation—represents a perfect example of a Kuhnian "paradigm shift." Kuhn, *Structure of Scientific Revolutions*.
32. The late nineteenth-century debate between "sanitarians" and "laboratory scientists" has been explored through a variety of national and colonial frames of reference. See Barnes, *Great Stink of Paris*; Tomes, *Gospel of Germs*; Worboys,

Spreading Germs; Latour, *Pasteurization of France*; Marcovich, "French Colonial Medicine and Colonial Rule."

33. Marcotte, *L'art de bâtir*, 169.
34. Marcotte, *L'art de bâtir*, 169, 202.
35. Marcotte, *L'art de bâtir*, 342–43.
36. Commune de la Goulette, "Règlement sanitaire," Title II, Article 10.
37. Commune de la Goulette, "Règlement sanitaire," Title II, Article 11.
38. Besson, *Traité élémentaire*, 40–44, 160.
39. Sebag, *Tunis*, 343.
40. Besson, *Traité élémentaire*, 156, 164.
41. Commune de la Goulette, "Règlement sanitaire," Title II, Article 15.
42. Marcotte, *L'art de bâtir*, 214.
43. Marcotte, *L'art de bâtir*, 216–17.
44. Marcotte, *L'art de bâtir*, 218–20, 243.
45. Avenue de la Marine, the main east-west thoroughfare in Tunis, was renamed Avenue Jules Ferry in 1900 and renamed again Avenue Habib Bourguiba after Tunisian independence in 1956.
46. Marcotte, *L'art de bâtir*, 197–98.
47. Daughton, *Empire Divided*, 13.
48. Commune de la Goulette, "Règlement sanitaire," Title II, Article 40.
49. Valensi and Wachtel, *Jewish Memories*, 43–44.
50. Cleere, "Victorian Dust Traps," 133.
51. Gross, "How Charles Nicolle of the Pasteur Institute."
52. Marcotte, *L'art de bâtir*, 396.
53. Conklin, *Mission to Civilize*, 217.
54. Hazbun, *Beaches, Ruins, Resorts*, 5.
55. For more on Orientalism in North Africa, see Benjamin, *Orientalist Aesthetics*; Kabbani, *Imperial Fictions*; Lowe, *Critical Terrains*.
56. The 1870 Crémieux Decree naturalized en masse the Jewish population of French Algeria, except for those in the northern Saharan villages of the M'zab.
57. Birnbaum, "French Jews and the 'Regeneration' of Algerian Jewry"; Zack, "French and Algerian Identity Formation"; Ansky, *Les Juifs d'Algérie*.
58. Sebag, *Histoire des Juifs de Tunisie*, 135–284.
59. Cole, "Anti-Semitism and the Colonial Situation"; on historical memories of the Crémieux Decree, see Katz, "Between Emancipation and Persecution."
60. For a similar example in French Algeria, see Cole, "Anti-Semitism and the Colonial Situation," 78.

61. For an in-depth discussion of the term "Arab Jew," see Gottreich, "Historicizing the Concept of Arab Jews in the Maghrib"; and Levy, "Historicizing the Concept of Arab Jews in the Mashriq."
62. Valensi and Wachtel, *Jewish Memories.*
63. This is an important observation noted by Valensi and Wachtel, *Jewish Memories,* 220.
64. Valensi and Wachtel, *Jewish Memories,* 219–20.
65. Daughton, *Empire Divided,* 21.
66. The interesting conflation of "race" and culture in colonial Algeria is explored in Lorcin, *Imperial Identities.*
67. Barbé, "Jewish-Muslim Syncretism," 115.
68. See Topalov, *Le logement en France*; Magri and Topalov, "L'habitat du salarié moderne en France."
69. Sanitary interventions in the Jewish hara are discussed in more detail in chapter 3.
70. Article 1 of the Arrêté du 29 novembre 1933 issued by the Vice Président de la Municipalité de Tunis.
71. The concept of "slumming" is explored in the American context in Heap, *Slumming.*
72. In the early twentieth century, the French considered "Arab" Muslims and Jews to be separate and distinct races, both from each other and from the French "race."
73. A. Green, *Tunisian Ulama,* 143.
74. Soulmagnon, *La loi tunisienne du 1er juillet,* 16.
75. Clancy-Smith, "Islam and the French Empire"; Sait and Lim, *Land, Law and Islam,* 3.
76. The modern debate over the alleged incompatibilities between shari'a law and "modern" property rights is explored in depth in Sait and Lim, *Land, Law and Islam.*
77. Perkins, *History of Modern Tunisia,* 45; Young, "Why Did the Torrens System Succeed?" 228.
78. Greg Taylor notes that the application of Torrens law in Tunisia may have been somewhat incomplete or subsequently modified. "Pierre Gebert, an acquaintance of this author who visited Tunisia in the 1980s as part of a review of the system of land titles in that country, reports that they system there could at best be said to have been inspired by the Torrens system, that indefeasibility is not offered by the legislation, and that title insurance flourishes there owing to confused land records and uncertainty as to boundaries. Unless there have been changes since the 1980s, therefore, Tunisia may no longer be a Torrens jurisdiction." Taylor, *Law of the Land,* fn 7.

79. *Habous* (also, Ar. *Waqf*) refers to the status of land under Islamic law whereby the property interest remains inalienable—the usufruct of such property accrues either to an individual family (private *habous*) or to a specified charity or religious organization (public *habous*). It is somewhat similar to the Anglo-American tradition of land held in trust. However, interference with *habous* is further complicated by the fact that the land is consecrated to Islam. (I use the French spelling *habous* for the Arabic, *ḣabs*, *ḣubus*, or *ḣubs*)
80. The descriptions and statistics are based on material in Sebag, *Tunis*. Many streets in Tunis were renamed after Tunisian independence in 1956. The suburb of Crémieuxville is absent from many maps of modern Tunis, and the hara is now commonly referred to by *tunisois* as El Hafsia. In addition, some of the sites on the modern map of Tunis do not correspond to the sites and names on colonial era maps as the neighborhoods have changed names or bled together. Franceville and El Omrane represent two such sites with mutated boundaries.
81. Chikly, *Tunis, Goulette, Marsa*, 67–70 (translation mine).
82. For more on racial and socioeconomic segregation in Algeria, see Prochaska, *Making Algeria French*, 153–79; Kalman, "Fascism and Algérianité."
83. *La Cagna*—a French slang word used by veterans of World War I trench warfare—means "shelter." It is derived from the Vietnamese word for house and was popularized in military parlance by veterans who had previously served in the French colonies in Southeast Asia. The protectorate used the slang term to designate the neighborhood reserved for French veterans.
84. For similar examples of the policing of "marginal whites" in the colonies and the notion that lower-class whites represented an enormous blow to the prestige of the imperial mission, see Stoler, *Carnal Knowledge*; and Cooper and Stoler, *Tensions of Empire*, pts. 1 and 2.
85. El Farabi (Abu Nasr al-Farabi) was a ninth-century scientist, intellectual, and philosopher. Amine Arrihaini (Amin al-Rihani) was an early twentieth-century Lebanese American writer and intellectual who was an early advocate of Arab nationalism. These figures would have been well-known to educated Muslims.
86. As previously mentioned, these notes and statistics come from Sebag, *Tunis*.
87. Lewis, *Divided Rule*, 108–18, 141. Lewis's book contains an entire chapter on the politics of cemeteries in French Tunisia. Le Pautremat and Ageron, *La politique musulmane de la France*, 90. These protests are referred to as the "streetcar riots." During the demonstrations against the surveying crew, a streetcar inadvertently struck a child in the confusion, which intensified public reaction against the survey.

88. Allen, *Cleansing the City*, 117, quoting Winter, *London's Teeming Streets*.
89. Records of the Tribunal mixte de Tunis, docket number 4580, dated January 5, 1901, held at Archives nationales de Tunisie (ANT), Série E, Carton 360, Dossier ½ (1939).
90. ANT, Série E, Carton 360, Dossier (1939). Letter from the Directeur de l'Administration Générale et Communale to the Secrétaire Général du Gouvernement Tunisien.
91. In 1936 the population of Tunis was 205,305 persons, of whom only 80,549 (39 percent) were Muslim. The remaining breakdown is as follows: 42,678 French, 49,878 Italians, 4,855 Maltese, and 27,345 Jews (Jews who were not French, Italian, or Maltese). Service Tunisien des Statistiques, *Annuaire statistique de la Tunisie* (Tunis, 1936).
92. Marçais, *L'Architecture musulmane d'Occident*; Marçais, *L'art musulman*.
93. Janet Abu-Lughod criticizes Marçais for not focusing on the *processes* that created the "Islamic city," which in her view were distinctions between Muslims and outsiders, gender segregation, and a laissez-faire system of property law. "Islamic City," 172.
94. For a complete analysis of the Orientalist view of the "Islamic city," see Gottriech, "Rethinking the 'Islamic City.'" See also Miller and Bertagnin, *Architecture and Memory of the Minority Quarter*.

3. Regenerating Space, Part 2

1. Eloy, *La Ville de Tunis à l'Exposition Coloniale Internationale*; Morton, *Hybrid Modernities*; Sherman, "Arts and Sciences of Colonialism."
2. Sebag, *Hara de Tunis*, 24–28.
3. Sebag, *Hara de Tunis*, 26.
4. Gottreich, *Mellah of Marrakesh*; Abu-Lughod, "Islamic City."
5. Antébi, *Les Missionaires juifs*; Slymovics, "Geographies of Jewish Tlemcen"; Rodrigue, *Images of Sephardi*; Laskier, *Alliance Israélite Universelle*.
6. Schroeter, "Jewish Quarter of the Moroccan City"; Schroeter, "Jewish Quarters in the Arab-Islamic Cities of the Ottoman Empire"; Gottreich, *Mellah of Marrakesh*; Miller et al., "Inscribing Minority Space"; S. G. Miller, "Apportioning Sacred Space in a Moroccan City."
7. Sebag, *Hara de Tunis*; Abdelkafi, *La Médina de Tunis*.
8. Clancy-Smith, *Mediterraneans*; Clancy-Smith, "'Making It' in Pre-colonial Tunis"; Larguèche, *Les ombres de Tunis*.
9. Cohen and Johnson, *Filth*, xx.

10. Schreier, "From Jewish Regeneration to Colonialism."
11. Hyman, *Jews of Modern France*, 53–73; Hyman, *From Dreyfus to Vichy*, 132–43.
12. Rodrigue, *Images of Sephardi*, 7–10; Antébi, *Les Missionaires juifs*, 11–17.
13. Hyman, *Jews of Modern France*, 116; Hyman, *From Dreyfus to Vichy*, 28–29.
14. Robert, "Nos édiles," 57, reprinted in Fijalkow, *Construction des ilôts insalubres*, 154; N. Green, *Pletzl of Paris*; Boyarin, *Polish Jews in Paris*.
15. Schneider, *Quality and Quantity*, 11–54; Klaus, *Every Child a Lion*, 14–31.
16. Badini-Jourdin, "Rapports et documents," *Bulletin municipal officiel de la Ville de Paris* (BMOVP), no. 108 (1909): 2, reprinted in Fijalkow, *Construction des îlots insalubres*, 155; for a history of the roots of the danger of "sordid foreigners," see Chevalier, *Labouring Classes and Dangerous Classes in Paris*, 293–309.
17. Badini-Jourdin, "Debats au Conseil Municipal de Paris du 8 décembre 1911," BMOVP SU 1782 (1911), reprinted in Fijalkow, *Construction des îlots insalubres*, 156.
18. Historian Peter Jackson has argued that there is a long-standing tradition of viewing French history as a continuous narrative of decline, fall, and renewal. The history of the Third Republic is often seen as one of slow decline before the defeat of 1940. See Jackson, "Post-War Politics." The Third Republic was fraught with political and social problems from its inception. These tensions are explored in N. Jordan, *Popular Front and Central Europe*; Duroselle, *Politique étrangère de la France*; Berstein, *La France des années 30*; Adamthwaite, *Grandeur and Misery*.
19. An article in *Le Journal*, 15 octobre 1920, cited in Hartmann, "Les étrangers au quartier Saint Gervais," 143–57, reprinted in Fijalkow, *Construction des îlots insalubres*,156.
20. Lauzel, "Un étrange quartier," 777–93.
21. Lauzel, "Un étrange quartier," 777–93.
22. "Cloaque de Paris," reprinted in Fijalkow, *Construction des îlots insalubres*, 166.
23. Marcotte, *L'art de bâtir*, 226–27.
24. Marcotte, *L'art de bâtir*, 226.
25. D. Jordan, "Haussmann and Haussmannisation," 87–113, 89.
26. Laloum, "Entre aryanisation et déportations"; Adler, *Jews of Paris and the Final Solution*, 23, 29.
27. "Rehousing" was the Vichy euphemism for the roundup (*les rafles*) and sequestration of Jews in "transit camps," such as the infamous Drancy camp outside Paris. Sixty-five thousand Jews were sent from Drancy to Auschwitz, where 62,000 of them, including 6,000 children, were murdered.
28. Clancy-Smith, *Mediterraneans*, 200.

29. Perpetua, *Geografia della Reggenza di Tunisi*, 173; Ganiage, *La crise des finances tunisiennes et l'ascension des juifs de Tunis*, 154; Larguèche, *Les ombres de Tunis*, 68–70, 299.
30. Clancy-Smith, *Mediterraneans*, 199–246.
31. Clancy-Smith, *Mediterraneans*, 209–11.
32. Letter from Résident général of the Tunisian Protectorate, René Millet, to the Quai d'Orsay dated January 14, 1899, Archives diplomatiques du Ministère des Affaires Étrangères (ADMAE), Israélites de Tunisie, folder II.
33. Sebag, *Histoire des Juifs de Tunisie*, 153.
34. The anticolonial voices in parliament were led by *revanchistes*, such as Georges Clemenceau, Jean Jaurès, and Maurice Barrès, who viewed colonial meddling as a distraction from France's primary threat: a unified Germany. Ironically, it was those who most embodied the "republican" spirit, such as Léon Gambetta and Jules Ferry, who sought to expand France's colonial empire. For more on the Third Republic, see Fortescue, *Third Republic in France*; Sowerwine, *France since 1870*.
35. Service Tunisien des Statistiques, *Annuaire statistique de la Tunisie* (Tunis, 1946), in Hagège and Zarca, "Les Juifs et la France," 12.
36. Service Tunisien des Statistiques, in Hagège and Zarca, "Les Juifs et la France," 17.
37. Sebag, *Histoire des Juifs de Tunisie*, 157–58.
38. "Destour" is the Arabic word (*dustūr*) for "constitution."
39. Sebag, *Histoire des Juifs de Tunisie*, 161–62. The sensitivity of the issue is demonstrated by the fact that the law was issued by the president of France, not the resident general via beylical decree as was customary.
40. Perkins, *History of Modern Tunisia*, 91.
41. Service Tunisien des Statistiques, in Hagège and Zarca, "Les Juifs et la France," 17.
42. Bessis, *La Méditerranée fasciste*, 34–41; Priestly, *France Overseas*, 188–99.
43. Djebali, "Ethnicity and Power in North Africa," 144.
44. Service Tunisien des Statistiques, in Hagège and Zarca, "Les Juifs et la France," 17.
45. Lewis, *Divided Rule*, 118, citing El Ghoul, *Naturalisation et Nationalisme en Tunisie*, 37.
46. On the inherent inconsistencies of the Crémieux Decree, see Schreier, "Napoleon's Long Shadow," 77–103.
47. Haim Saadoun has written extensively on Zionism in Tunisia in Hebrew. For example, Saadoun, "Zionism in Tunisia"; see also Saadoun, "L'influence du sionisme," 219–29; Perkins, *History of Modern Tunisia*, 46.

48. Perkins, *History of Modern Tunisia*, 93, citing Majhoubi, *Les Origines du mouvement national en Tunisie*, 563.
49. Perkins, *History of Modern Tunisia*, 94–95.
50. Cohen-Hadria, *Du Protectorat français à l'Indépendance*.
51. Kazdaghli, "L'évolution organisationnelle du mouvement communiste en Tunisie."
52. Gottreich, *Mellah of Marrakesh*, 2–4; Deshen, *Mellah Society*, 13–29; Kenbib, *Juifs et Musulmans au Maroc*, 50–57; Abu-Lughod, "Islamic City," 165–67.
53. Sebag, *Hara de Tunis*, 13.
54. *Bulletin municipal officiel de la Ville de Tunis* (BMOVT), 21 année, no. 78 (1930). The likelihood that the Jewish statistic is primarily made up of hara Jews is bolstered by the fact that many of the Jews who had left the hara were counted as French. The death rate of French *tunisois* during the same period was 16.36 per 1,000.
55. BMOVT, 16 année, no. 56 (1924); BMOVT, 16 année, no. 58 (1924); BMOVT, 19 année, no. 69 (1927); BMOVT, 19 année, no. 71 (1927): BMOVT, 20 année, no. 74 (1928); and BMOVT, 21 année, no. 78 (1930). My calculations include the following as infectious diseases: typhoid fever, typhus, measles, whooping cough, diphtheria, cholera, tuberculosis, pneumonia, and infant diarrhea.
56. Nash, *Inescapable Ecologies*, 88.
57. Even a cursory examination of the AIU's archives in Paris demonstrates that the opinions of, and differences between, instructors and principals of alliance schools in Tunisia were varied and diverse. But for the most part, those affiliated with the alliance joined the call for hygienic intervention in the hara.
58. Marcotte, *L'art de bâtir*, 396, 230.
59. Royer, *L'Urbanisme aux colonies et dans les pays tropicaux*, 54.
60. The idea that Jews could be "regenerated" has a long history in France. Its most famous advocate was Abbé Grégoire (Henri Grégoire). For a discussion of the evolution of "regeneration" ideology, see Schreier, *From Jewish Regeneration*.
61. BMOVT, 16 année, no. 56 (1924).
62. Jews were 13 percent of the population of Tunis in 1926. However, this statistic does not include the estimated 17 percent of Tunisian Jews who were counted as French or Italian citizens (most of whom lived in Tunis). Attal and Sitbon, *Regards sur les juifs de Tunisie*, 291–95.
63. The report divided Tunis's population into seven categories: French, Italian, Anglo-Maltese, other Europeans, Tunisian Jews, those who held *habous*, and indigenous Muslims. I have combined the statistics for those who held *habous* with the statistics for indigenous Muslims because *habous* could only be held by the latter.

64. ANT, "Internal memo for the Secretary General of the Governent from the Delegate Vice-President of the Municipality of Tunis," Série E, Carton 621, Dossier 14, Sous-dossier 220.
65. "Rapport du Directeur des Travaux de la Ville au Conseil Municipal le 6 août 1936," *BMOVT*, 29 année, no. 107 (1937).
66. *BMOVT*, 28 année, no. 105 (1936).
67. "Rapport du Directeur des Travaux de la Ville au Conseil Municipal," *BMOVT*, 29 année, no. 108 (1938).
68. *BMOVT*, 28 année, no. 107 (1937).
69. "Session Extraordinaire du Séance du 18 janvier 1939," *BMOVT*, 31 année, no. 115 (1939).
70. "Session Extraordinaire du Séance du 18 janvier 1939,"
71. "Rapport du Directeur des Travaux de la Ville au Conseil Municipal," *BMOVT*, 31 année, no. 115 (1939).
72. "Session Extraordinaire du Séance du 18 janvier 1939."
73. Ross, *Fast Cars, Clean Bodies*, 71–104.
74. Barnes, *Great Stink of Paris*, 8.
75. The same connection between modernity and assimilationist housing for Jews was made in interwar Algeria. See Cole, "Anti-Semitism and the Colonial Situation," 86.
76. "Débat entre le Directeur des Travaux de la Ville et le Conseil Municipal." *BMOVT*, 26 année, no. 95 (1934).
77. Cole, "Anti-Semitism and the Colonial Situation," 78.
78. "Séance du Conseil Municipal au 18 novembre 1935," *BMOVT*, 27 année, no. 102 (1936).
79. *BMOVT*, 27 année, no. 102 (1936).
80. *BMOVT*, 27 année, no. 102 (1936).
81. Conklin, "Redefining 'Frenchness'"; Stoler, *Carnal Knowledge*, 79–111.
82. Schechter, *Obstinate Hebrews*; Graetz, *Jews in Nineteenth Century France*; Berkovitz, *Shaping of Jewish Identity*; Albert, *Modernization of French Jewry*; Hyman, *Jews of Modern France*; Hyman, *From Dreyfus to Vichy*; Hyman, *Emancipation of the Jews*.
83. Wright, "Tradition in the Service of Modernity," 294.
84. Miller et al., "Inscribing Minority Space."
85. Larguèche, *Les ombres de Tunis*, 299.
86. Barbé, "Jewish-Muslim Syncretism," 113–17.
87. Hyman, *From Dreyfus to Vichy*, 39–43; Hyman, *Jews of Modern France*, 38, 74–75.
88. Rabinow, *French Modern*, 297–301, 325–26; Çelik, *Urban Forms and Colonial Confrontations*, 8; Wright, *Politics of Design*, 10, 28, 54; Betts, *Assimilation and Association*.

89. Marcotte, *L'art de bâtir*, 392.

4. Regenerating Youth

1. For an excellent exploration of post–World War II relations between Muslims and Jews and their relation to France, see Mandel, *Muslims and Jews in France.*
2. Rodrigue, *Images of Sephardi*, 7–10; Laskier, *Alliance Israélite Universelle*, 25–54; Silberman, "Investigation of the Schools," 56–72.
3. Archives de l'Alliance Israélite Universelle (AAIU), *Instructions générales*, in Rodrigue, *Images of Sephardi*, 44.
4. AAIU, *Instructions générales.*
5. Conklin, *Mission to Civilize*, 5–6.
6. "Tableau des écoles," *Bulletin de l'Alliance Israélite Universelle. Mensuel 1913*, 75–115, in Laskier, "Aspects of the Activities of the Alliance Israelite Universelle," 167. For more statistics on the AIU's Mediterranean network, see Rodrigue, *De l'Instruction à l'Emancipation.*
7. AAIU, Iran I.F.1, in Rodrigue, *Images of Sephardi*, 52.
8. Letter Tunis, 6 February 1908, AAIU, Tunisie II.C.5, in Rodrigue, *Images of Sephardi*, 78.
9. AAIU, *Instructions générales pour les professeurs* (Paris, 1903), 63.
10. Presner, *Muscular Judaism*, 117, quoting Nye, *Crime, Madness, and Politics in Modern France*, 328.
11. Shanahan, *Evolution of Darwinism*; Bowler, *Eclipse of Darwinism.*
12. Pick, *Faces of Degeneration*; Goldstein, *Console and Classify.*
13. For the formation of Lamarckian and neo-Larmarckian ideas of trait heritability in the French context, see Conklin, *In the Museum of Man*, 33, 44–45.
14. "We find another explanation in the changing conception of poverty, from the idea of poverty as a condition affecting the individual and subject to the immediate influence of sanitary and philanthropic intervention, to the idea of poverty as a sociobiological phenomenon bred into the population and over which reformers had little control." Allen, *Cleansing the City*, 116.
15. Cheyette and Valman, *Image of the Jew in European Liberal Culture*; Gilman, *Jew's Body*; Kruger, *Spectral Jew.*
16. Dubow, *Scientific Racism in Modern South Africa.*
17. For a compelling description of the discursive power of the Muscular Judaism movement—medically, politically, and socially—see Presner, *Muscular Judaism.*
18. Falk, "Zionism and the Biology of the Jews," 587–607.
19. Nordau, *Degeneration*; Herzl, *Der Judenstaat.*
20. Marrus, *Politics of Assimilation*, 245–46, 267, 282–85.

21. For a general overview of early Zionism in the Maghrib, see Laskier, "Evolution of Zionist Activity," 205–36.
22. For more on the active Jewish press in Tunisia, see Attal, *La Presse Périodique Juive*; Sebag, *Histoire des Juifs de Tunisie*, 23.
23. Snouissi, "Aux origines du mouvement sioniste en Tunisie"; Kassab, "La communauté israélite de Tunisie."
24. Sebag, *Histoire des Juifs de Tunisie*, 20.
25. Sebag, *Histoire des Juifs de Tunisie*, 23.
26. See generally, Attal, *La Presse Périodique Juive*.
27. Sebag, *Histoire des Juifs de Tunisie*, 18–9.
28. Tobi, "Flāḥ, Shalom."
29. Graetz, *Jews in Nineteenth Century France*.
30. Fellous, *Juifs et Musulmans en Tunisie*, 209.
31. ANT, Série E, Carton 262, Dossier 21.
32. Udovitch and Valensi, *Last Arab Jews*, 21.
33. Saadoun, "L'influence du sionisme," 223. Tensions between the Jewish and Muslim communities were heightened by the 1929 events in Palestine, tensions between Zionists and Destourians even more so.
34. Saadoun, "L'influence du sionisme," 223.
35. Saadoun, "L'influence du sionisme," 224.
36. ANT, Série E, Carton 509, Dossier 154.
37. ANT, Série E, Carton 509, Dossier169.
38. AAIU, Israel II.C.10, in Rodrigue, *Images of Sephardi*, 245–46.
39. AAIU, Israel II.C.10, in Rodrigue, *Images of Sephardi*, 245–46.
40. AAIU, France XVII.F.28, in Rodrigue, *Images of Sephardi*, 133–34.
41. Kuperminc, "Le Regard," 347–56.
42. Kuperminc, "Le Regard," 347–56.
43. ANT, Série E, Carton 509, Dossier 155.
44. Antébi, *Les Missionaires juifs*, 197–98.
45. Presner, *Muscular Judiasm*, 123, quoting *Die Jüdische Turnzeitung*, 1900, 1:1.
46. Letter from Veron to AIU, May 2, 1930, AAIU, Etats-Unis II. A7 in Antébi, *Les Missionaires juifs*, 330.
47. Antébi, *Les Missionaires juifs*, 124.
48. See generally Presner, *Muscular Judaism*; Nye, "Degeneration, Neurasthenia, and the Culture of Sport," 51–68.
49. *L'Aurore*, "Les Sports," January 29, 1934. "Dès le gong annonçant le début du premier round, tel un tigre sur sa proie, 'l'enfant des souks' se jeta sur son adversaire et le cribla de ses poings. Sous le dynamisme puissant du valeureux

tunisien, Huat resta quelque instant pantois; se rendant compte de la réelle valeur de son adversaire."

50. Rauch, *Boxe, violence du XXe siècle*, 27.
51. Letter of August 30, 1932, sent by the delegate of the resident general to the minister of foreign affairs, ADMAE, Tunisie 1917–1940: C. 381.
52. Chikly, *Tunis, Goulette, Marsa*, 20–21.
53. Letter from M. Cohen to Alliance headquarters, AAIU, Tunisie I.G.3, in Rodrigue, *Images of Sephardi*, 255.
54. Tunisia never witnessed anti-Jewish activity on the scale of that seen in Constantine, Algeria, or French Morocco. The origins of the rioting that occurred throughout the Maghrib between 1933 and 1934 are difficult to pinpoint, as explained in Laskier, *North African Jewry*, 56–58.

5. Regenerating Women

1. More information on Habiba M'sika can be found in Faivre d'Arcier, *Habiba Messika*; and Hamrouni, *Habiba M'skia*. As was the case with Habiba's life, these accounts cross the boundaries of fiction and reality with relative ease.
2. Ehrenreich and English, *Witches, Midwives, and Nurses*; S. A. Miller, *Medieval Monstrosity and the Female Body*; Laqueur, *Making Sex*.
3. Starr, *Social Transformation of American Medicine*; Vogel and Rosenberg, *Therapeutic Revolution*; Jacob, *Cultural Meaning of the Scientific Revolution*; Silver, *Ascent of Science*.
4. Tomes, *Gospel of Germs*.
5. Hyman, *Gender and Assimilation*; Simonsen, *Making Home Work*; Kaplan, *Making of the Jewish Middle Class*; Litt, *Medicalized Motherhood*; Adams, *Poverty, Charity, and Motherhood*.
6. Stoler, *Carnal Knowledge*; Cooper and Stoler, *Tensions of Empire*; Clancy-Smith and Gouda, *Domesticating the Empire*; Hunt, *Colonial Lexicon*; Briggs, *Reproducing Empire*.
7. Muraud, *L'hygiene dans la Republique*; Baldwin, *Contagion and the State in Europe*; Coleman, *Death Is a Social Disease*.
8. Nye, *Crime, Madness, and Politics*, 328.
9. Cooper and Stoler, *Tensions of Empire*; Stoler, *Race and the Education of Desire*; Stoler, *Carnal Knowledge*; Clancy-Smith and Gouda, *Domesticating the Empire*.
10. Said, *Orientalism*; Arnold, *Colonizing the Body*; Bhabha, *Location of Culture*; Dirks, *Castes of Mind*. In the Maghribi context, see Benjamin, *Orientalist Aesthetics*; Kabbani, *Imperial Fictions*; Lowe, *Critical Terrains*.
11. Schechter, *Obstinate Hebrews*; Graetz, *Jews in Nineteenth Century France*; Berkovitz, *Shaping of Jewish Identity*; Albert, *Modernization of French Jewry*.

12. Grégoire, *Essai sur la régénération*. For more on this topic, Sepinwall, *Abbé Grégoire*; Necheles, *Abbé Grégoire*.
13. Rodrigue, *French Jews, Turkish Jews*; Rodrigue, *Images of Sephardi*; Laskier, *Alliance Israélite Universelle*; Chouraqui, *L'Alliance Israélite universelle*.
14. Service Tunisien des Statistiques, in Hagège and Zarca, "Les Juifs et la France," 17.
15. Djebali, "Ethnicity and Power in North Africa," 144. The *loi Morinaud* of 1923 eased the requirements even more.
16. Hyman, *Gender and Assimilation*, 13.
17. Hyman, *Gender and Assimilation*, 13.
18. Schroeter, *Merchants of Essaouira*; Schroeter, *Sultan's Jew*.
19. Gilman, *Difference and Pathology*; Gilman, *Jew's Body*.
20. Hesse-Wartegg, *Tunis, Land und Leute*, 101; Maltzan, *Reise in den Regenschaften Tunis und Tripolis*, 27–28, 40–41, 73, 97–98.
21. AAIU, *Instructions générales*, 75–78, in Rodrigue, *Images of Sephardi*, 38–39.
22. Conklin, *Mission to Civilize*, 5–6.
23. Vassel, *Le Juif Tunisien*, 3.
24. Voligny, *À Tunis*, 78.
25. Hyman, *From Dreyfus to Vichy*, 39–43; Hyman, *Emancipation of the Jews*; Hyman, *Jews of Modern France*, 38, 74–5; N. Green, *Pletzl of Paris*.
26. Hyman, *Jews of Modern France*, 115, 119, 122.
27. Shah, *Contagious Divides*, 77–79.
28. Sarfati, *Tounis "El Khadra,"* 52, 53.
29. Manderson, "Shaping Reproduction," 28.
30. Hyman, *Jews of Modern France*, 131. The growing Zionist movement in Tunisia represented the singular challenge to bourgeois Frenchification schemes, as demonstrated by Saadoun, "Zionism in Tunisia."
31. Clarke, "Population of Tunisia," 366.
32. Taïeb, "Évolution et comportement démographiques," 957.
33. Accampo, *Industrialization, Family Life, and Class Relations*. Accampo argues that working-class women began to limit family size much earlier than hitherto believed by historians.
34. ANT, Série E, Carton 509, Dossier 19.
35. ANT, Série E, Carton 509, Dossier 19.
36. Voligny, *À Tunis*, 76.
37. AAIU, France XIV. F. 25, in Rodrigue, *Images of Sephardi*, 90–91.
38. Burnet, *Enquête sur l'alimentation en Tunisie*.
39. AAIU, 2 B 12–14, Carton 149, Bobine 33.

40. AAIU, France XIV. F. 25, in Rodrigue, *Images of Sephardi*, 90–91.
41. ANT, Série SG, Sous-series SG2, Carton 63, Dossiers 31 and 42bis; ANT, Série E, Carton 509, Dossiers 48 and 169.
42. ANT, Série E, Carton 509, Dossier 19.
43. ANT, Série SG/SG 95, Carton 34, Dossier 27. Letter from Dr. Dupoux, Inspector of Social Hygiene and Preventive Medicine to the Director-General of the Interior dated 15 October 1936.
44. ANT, Série SG/SG 95, Carton 34, Dossier 27.
45. Zarca, *Une enfance juive tunisoise*, 78; Voligny, *À Tunis*, 79.
46. AAIU, France XIV. F. 25, in Rodrigue, *Images of Sephardi*, 90–91.
47. AAIU, France XIV. F. 25, in Rodrigue, *Images of Sephardi*, 90–91.
48. ANT, Série E, Carton 509, Dossier 19.
49. Vassel, *Le Juif Tunisien*, 3.
50. AAIU, Tunisie XXIV.E.198a. Letter from Headmaster Albert Saguès to the Headquarters of the AIU in Paris, dated October 1912.
51. Voligny, *À Tunis*, 77. For more on the AIU's influence on women, see Land, "Corresponding Lives;" Rodrigue, *Images of Sephardi*; Laskier, *Alliance Israélite Universelle.*
52. Sarfati, *Tounis "El Khadra,"* 47–48.
53. Zarca, *Une enfance juive tunisoise*, 110.
54. Lorcin, "Teaching Women and Gender," 294–96.
55. *BMOVT*, 21 année, no. 78 (1930).
56. This definition of "medicalized maternity" is taken from Jolly, "Introduction," 6.
57. Valensi and Wachtel, *Jewish Memories*, 219–20.
58. Dinguizli, *Réformes hygiéniques.*
59. Gaumer, *L'organisation*, 155.
60. Gaumer, *L'organisation*, 155, 221.
61. Jolly, "Introduction."
62. Dinguizli, *Réformes hygiéniques.*
63. Archives diplomatiques de Nantes, Protectorat Tunisie, bobine 2MI 399, vol. 1957, dossier 1, citing J. Sclema, *Sur la nécessité d'une réglementation rigoureuse de l'exercice de la profession des sages-femmes en Tunisie.*
64. Dinguizli, *Réformes hygiéniques.*
65. *Journal Officiel de la République Tunisienne* (*JORT*), 1892, 364–65. The remaining fifty-nine physicians were primarily Muslims who were locally trained and "tolerated" (*médicins tolérés*) by the regime.
66. Gaumer, *L'organisation*, 216.

67. Gaumer, *L'organisation*, 18, citing Chevalier, *Le problême démographique nord-africain*. Of this 2.1 million, 54,000 were French-born colonists, another 54,000 were indigenous Jews, and 1.98 million were indigenous Muslims.
68. Gaumer, *L'organisation*, 216.
69. See also Nahum, *Le médicine française et les Juifs*.
70. Gaumer, *L'organisation*, 232–33, citing Malinas and Tostivint, "Mutualité coöperative et projet général d'assistance médicale indigène," 480–515.
71. Gaumer, *L'organisation*, 154, 220.
72. Gaumer, *L'organisation*, 216, citing "Dossier Affaire Pinner," in ADMAE, series Tunisie, 1930–1940, no. 682, 7–13.
73. Gaumer, *L'organisation*, 216, citing "Dossier Médecins Israélites allemands" and "Dossier, 15 juillet et 23 novembre 1933," in ADMAE, series Tunisie, 1930–1940, no. 682, 33 and 34.
74. Berstein, *La France des années 30*; Winock, *Histoire de l'extrême droite en France*; Winock, *Nationalisme, fascism et antisémitisme en France*.
75. Gallagher, *Medicine and Power*.
76. Report from the Direction générale de l'Intérieur, *Monographies des Services* (Bourg: Victor Berthod, 1931).
77. Gaumer, *L'organisation*, 34, citing David and Nacasch, *Bulletin économique et social de la Tunisie*, 11.
78. For example, Achterberg, *Woman as Healer*; Ehrenreich and English, *For Her Own Good*; Ulrich, *Life of Martha Ballard*.

BIBLIOGRAPHY

Abdelkafi, Jellal. *La Médina de Tunis*. Paris: Presses du CNRS, 1986.

Abi-Mershed, Osama. *Apostles of Modernity: Saint-Simonians and the Civilizing Mission in Algeria*. Palo Alto CA: Stanford University Press, 2010.

Abu-Lughod, Janet. "The Islamic City: Historic Myth, Islamic Essence, and Contemporary Relevance." *International Journal of Middle East Studies* 19 (May 1987): 155–76.

Accampo, Elinor. *Industrialization, Family Life, and Class Relations: Saint-Chamond, 1815–1914*. Berkeley: University of California Press, 1989.

Achterberg, Jeanne. *Woman as Healer*. Boston: Shambhala, 1991.

Adams, Christine. *Poverty, Charity, and Motherhood: Maternal Societies in Nineteenth-Century France*. Urbana: University of Illinois Press, 2010.

Adams, Julia, and Isaac Ariail Reed. "Culture in the Transitions to Modernity: Seven Pillars of a New Research Agenda." *Theory & Society* 40 (2011): 247–72.

Adamthwaite, A. *Grandeur and Misery: France's Bid for Power in Europe, 1914–1940*. London: Arnold, 1995.

Adler, Jacques. *The Jews of Paris and the Final Solution: Communal Response and Internal Conflicts, 1940–1944*. New York: Oxford University Press, 1987.

Albert, Phyllis Cohen. "Israelite and Jew: How Did Nineteenth-Century French Jews Understand Assimilation?" In *Assimilation and Community in European Jewry, 1815–1881*, edited by Jonathan Frankel and Steven Zipperstein, 88–109. Cambridge: Cambridge University Press, 1991.

———. *The Modernization of French Jewry: Consistory and Community in the Nineteenth Century*. Hanover NH: Brandeis University Press, 1977.

Aldrich, Robert. *Greater France: A History of French Overseas Expansion*. New York: Palgrave, 1996.

Allen, Michelle. *Cleansing the City: Sanitary Geographies in Victorian London*. Athens: Ohio University Press, 2007.

Amster, Ellen. *Medicine and the Saints: Science, Islam, and the Colonial Experience in Morocco, 1877–1956*. Austin: University of Texas, 2013.

Ansky, Michel. *Les Juifs d'Algérie: Du decret Crémieux à la Libération.* Paris, 1950.

Antébi, Elizabeth. *Les Missionnaires juifs de la France, 1860–1939.* Paris: Calman-Levy, 1999.

Arnold, David. *Colonizing the Body: State Medicine and Epidemic Disease in Nineteenth-Century India.* Berkeley: University of California Press, 1993.

Attal, Robert. *La Presse Périodique Juive de l'Afrique du Nord.* Tel Aviv: Tel Aviv University Press, 1996.

Attal, Robert, and Claude Sitbon. *Regards sur les juifs de Tunisie.* Paris: Albin Michel, 1979.

Bahloul, Joelle. *The Architecture of Memory: A Jewish-Muslim Household in Colonial Algeria, 1937–1962.* Cambridge: Cambridge University Press, 1996.

Baldwin, Peter. *Contagion and the State in Europe, 1830–1930.* Cambridge: Cambridge University Press, 1999.

Barbé, Philippe. "Jewish-Muslim Syncretism and Intercommunity Cohabitation in the Writings of Albert Memmi," translated by Allan MacVicar. In *Jewish Culture and Society in North Africa,* edited by Emily Gottreich and Daniel Schroeter, 107–27. Bloomington: Indiana University Press, 2011.

Barnes, David S. *The Great Stink of Paris and the Nineteenth Century Struggle against Filth and Germs.* Baltimore: Johns Hopkins University Press, 2006.

Benbassa, Esther. *Histoire des Juifs de France.* Paris: Editions du Seuil, 1997.

Benjamin, Roger. *Orientalist Aesthetics, Art, Colonialism and French North Africa: 1880–1930.* Berkeley: University of California Press, 2003.

Berkovitz, Jay. *The Shaping of Jewish Identity in Nineteenth-Century France.* Detroit: Wayne State University Press, 1989.

Berstein, Serge. *La France des années 30.* Paris: Armand Collin, 2001.

Bessis, Juliette. *La Méditerranée fasciste: l'Italie mussolinienne et la Tunisie.* Paris: Editions Karthala, 1981.

Besson, Albert. *Traité élémentaire d'hygiene.* Paris: Librairie J.-B. Bailliere et fils, 1896.

Betts, Raymond. *Assimilation and Association in French Colonial Theory, 1890–1914.* New York: Columbia University Press, 1961.

Bhabha, Homi. *The Location of Culture.* New York: Routledge, 1994.

———. "Unpacking My Library . . . Again." In *The Post-colonial Question: Common Skies, Divided Horizons,* edited by Iain Chambers and Lidia Curti, 199–211. London: Routledge, 1996.

———. "Unsatisfied: Notes on Vernacular Cosmopolitanism." In *Text and Nation: Cross-Disciplinary Essays on Cultural and National Identities,* edited by Laura Garcia-Moreno and Peter C. Pfeiffer, 191–207. Columbia SC: Camden House, 1996.

Birnbaum, Pierre. "French Jews and the 'Regeneration' of Algerian Jewry." *Studies in Contemporary Jewry* 19 (2003): 88–95.

Blaut, James M. *The Colonizer's Model of the World: Geographical Diffusionism and Eurocentric History*. New York: Guildford, 1993.

Blumenbach, Johann, et al. *On the Natural Varieties of Mankind: De generis humani varietate nativa*. New York: Bergman, 1969.

Bowler, P. *The Eclipse of Darwinism: Anti-Darwinian Evolution Theories in the Decades around 1900*. Baltimore: Johns Hopkins University Press, 1983.

Boyarin, Jonathan. *Polish Jews in Paris: The Ethnography of Memory*. Bloomington: Indiana University Press, 1991.

Braunschvig, R. "Tunisia." In *E. J. Brill's First Encyclopedia of Islam, 1913–1936*. 8 vols. 1913. Reprint, Leiden: Brill, 1987.

Briggs, Laura. *Reproducing Empire: Race, Sex, Science and U.S. Imperialism in Puerto Rico*. Berkeley: University of California Press, 2002.

Brower, Benjamin C. *A Desert Named Peace: The Violence of France's Empire in the Algerian Sahara, 1844–1902*. New York: Columbia University Press, 2011.

Buffon, George-Louis de. *Natural History*. Vol. 4. London: J. S. Barr, 1792.

Buican, Denis. "Sur le développement de la génétique classique en France." *Revue du synthèse* (1973): 240–41.

Burnet, Étienne. *Enquête sur l'alimentation en Tunisie*. Tunis: Imprimerie Bascone et Muscat, 1939.

Canestri, R. "Relationship between Ideology and Science." *Forum (Genova)* 9, no. 2 (April–June 1999): 183–90.

Catalan, Tullia. "The Ambivalence of a Port-City: The Jews of Trieste from the 19th to the 20th Century." *Quest Issues in Contemporary Jewish History. Journal of Fondazione CDEC*, no. 2 (October 2, 2011). www.quest-cdecjournal.it/focus.php?id=232.

Catro-Gómez, Santiago. "The Social Sciences, Epistemic Violence, and the Problem of the 'Invention of the Other.'" In *Unbecoming Modern: Colonialism, Modernity, Colonial Modernities*, edited by Saurabh Dube and Ishita Banerjee-Dube, 211–27. New Delhi: Social Science Press, 2006.

Celestin, Roger, and Eliane DalMolin. *France from 1851 to the Present: Universalism in Crisis*. London: Palgrave, 2007.

Çelik, Zeynep. *Urban Forms and Colonial Confrontations: Algiers under French Rule*. Berkeley: University of California Press, 1997.

Chartier, Roger. *Cultural History: Between Practices and Representations*. Edited by Lydia G. Cochrane. Ithaca NY: Cornell University Press, 1988.

Chevalier, L. *Le problême démographique nord-africain*. Paris: Presses universitaires de France, 1947.

Chevalier, Louis. *Labouring Classes and Dangerous Classes in Paris during the First Half of the Nineteenth Century*. London: Routledge & Kegan Paul, 1973.

Cheyette, Bryan, and Nadia Valman. *The Image of the Jew in European Liberal Culture, 1789–1914*. London: Vallentine Mitchell, 2004.

Chikly, Gilbert. *Tunis, Goulette, Marsa: Aux yeux du souvenir*. Montmorency: Edition Gilbert Chikly, 1999.

Choate, Mark I. "Identity Politics and Political Perception in the European Settlement of Tunisia: The French Colony versus the Italian Colony." *French Colonial History* 8 (2007): 97–109.

Chouraqui, Andre. *L'Alliance Israélite universelle et la renaissance juive contemporaines, 1860–1960, cent ans d'histoire*. Paris: Presses universitaires de France, 1965.

Clancy-Smith, Julia. "Gender in the City: Women, Migration, and Contested Spaces in Tunis, c. 1830–1881." In *Africa's Urban Past*, edited by David Anderson and Richard Rathbone, 189–204. Oxford: James Currey and Heinemann, 2000.

———. "Islam and the French Empire in North Africa." In *Islam and the European Empires*, edited by David Motadel, 90–111. Oxford: Oxford University Press, 2014.

———. "'Making It' in Pre-colonial Tunis: Migration, Work, and Poverty in a Mediterranean Port-City, c. 1815–1870." In *Subalterns and Social Protest: History from Below in the Middle East and North Africa*, edited by Stephanie Cronin, 213–36. London: Routledge, 2007.

———. *Mediterraneans: North Africa and Europe in an Age of Migration, 1800–1900*. Berkeley: University of California Press, 2011.

———, ed. *North Africa, Islam and the Mediterranean World: From the Almoravids to the Algerian War*. London: Frank Cass, 2001.

Clancy-Smith, Julia, and Frances Gouda, eds. *Domesticating the Empire: Race, Gender, and Family Life in French and Dutch Colonialism*. Charlottesville: University of Virginia Press, 1998.

Clarke, John I. "The Population of Tunisia: An Example of Contact between Modern Civilization and the Moslem World." *Economic Geography* 28, no. 4 (October 1952): 366.

Cleere, Eileen. "Victorian Dust Traps." In *Filth: Dirt, Disgust, and Modern Life*, edited by William A. Cohen and Ryan Johnson, 133–55. Minneapolis: University of Minnesota Press, 2004.

Cohen, David. *Le Parler Arabe des Juifs de Tunis: textes et documents linguistiques et ethnographiques*. Paris: Mouton, 1964.

———. *La Promotion des Juifs en France à l'époque du second empire (1852–1870)*. Aix-Marseille: Université de Provence, 1980.

Cohen, Phyllis Albert. "Israelite and Jew: How Did Nineteenth-Century French Jews Understand Assimilation?" In *Assimilation and Community in European*

Jewry, 1815–1881, edited by Jonathan Frankel and Steven Zipperstein, 88–109. Cambridge: Cambridge University Press, 1991.

Cohen, William A., and Ryan Johnson, eds. *Filth: Dirt, Disgust, and Modern Life.* Minneapolis: University of Minnesota Press, 2004.

Cohen-Hadria, Élie. *Du Protectorat français à l'Indépendance tunisien (souvenirs d'un témoin socialiste)*. Nice: Université de Nice, 1977.

Cole, Joshua. "Anti-Semitism and the Colonial Situation in Interwar Algeria: The Anti-Jewish Riots in Constantine, August 1934." In *The French Colonial Mind*, vol. 2, edited by Martin Thomas, 77–111. Lincoln: University of Nebraska Press, 2011.

Coleman, William. *Death Is a Social Disease: Public Health and Political Economy in Early Industrial France.* Madison: University of Wisconsin Press, 1982.

Conklin, Alice. *In the Museum of Man: Race, Anthropology, and Empire in France, 1850–1950.* Ithaca NY: Cornell University Press, 2013.

———. *Mission to Civilize: The Republican Idea of Empire in France and West Africa, 1895–1930.* Palo Alto CA: Stanford University Press, 1997.

———. "Redefining 'Frenchness': France and West Africa." In *Domesticating the Empire: Race, Gender, and Family Life in French and Dutch Colonialism*, edited by Julia Clancy-Smith and Frances Gouda, 65–83. Charlottesville: University Press of Virginia, 1998.

Conry, Yvette. *L'Introduction du darwinisme en France au XIXe siècle.* Paris: Vrin, 1974.

Cooper, Frederick. *Colonialism in Question: Theory, Knowledge, and History.* Berkeley: University of California Press, 2005.

Cooper, Frederick, and Ann Laura Stoler, eds. *Tensions of Empire: Colonial Cultures in a Bourgeois World.* Berkeley: University of California Press, 1997.

Darwin, Charles. *De l'origine des espèces ou Des loi du progrès chez les êtres organisées.* Translated by Clémence Royer. Paris: Guillaumin et Cie., 1862.

Daughton, J. P. *An Empire Divided: Religion, Republicanism, and the Making of French Colonialism, 1880–1940.* Oxford: Oxford University Press, 2008.

Davis, Diana K. *Resurrecting the Granary of Rome: Environmental History and French Colonial Expansion in North Africa.* Athens: Ohio University Press, 2007.

Dedet, Jean-Pierre. *Les Institute Pasteur d'outre-mer: cent vingt ans de microbiologie française dans le monde.* Paris: L'Harmattan, 2000.

Del Piano, Lorenzo. *La penetrazione italiana in Tunisia, 1861–1881.* Padua: CEDAM, 1964.

Deshen, Shlomo. *Mellah Society: Jewish Community Life in Sherifian Morocco.* Chicago: University of Chicago Press, 1989.

Dewhurst, Mary Lewis. *Divided Rule: Sovereignty and Empire in Colonial Tunisia, 1881–1938.* Berkeley: University of California Press, 2014.

Dinguizli, Béchir. *Réformes hygiéniques, Rapport à la Commission d'hygiène*. Tunis: Imprimerie de la Presse, 1919.

Dirks, Nicholas. *Castes of Mind: Colonialism and the Making of Modern India*. Princeton NJ: Princeton University Press, 2001.

Djebali, Taoufik. "Ethnicity and Power in North Africa: Tunisia, Algeria and Morocco." In *Race and Nation: Ethnic Systems in the Modern World*, edited by Paul Spikard, 135–54. London: Routledge, 2005.

Dodds, Jerrilynn. *The Arts of Intimacy: Christians, Jews, and Muslims in the Making of Castilian Culture*. New Haven CT: Yale University Press, 2009.

Dube, Saurabh. *Stiches on Time: Colonial Textures and Postcolonial Tangles*. Durham NC: Duke University Press, 2004.

Dube, Saurabh, and Ishita Banerjee-Dube, eds. *Unbecoming Modern: Colonialism, Modernity, Colonial Modernities*. New Delhi: Social Science Press, 2006.

Dubin, Lois C. *The Port Jews of Habsburg Trieste: Absolutist Politics and Enlightenment Culture*. Palo Alto CA: Stanford University Press, 1999.

———. "Researching Port Jews and Port Jewries: Trieste and Beyond." In *Port Jews: Jewish Communities in Cosmopolitan Maritime Trading Centres, 1550–1950*, edited by David Cesarani, 47–58. London: Frank Cass, 2002.

Dubow, Saul. *Scientific Racism in Modern South Africa*. Cambridge: Cambridge University Press, 1995.

Duroselle, J.-B. *Politique étrangère de la France: la decadence*. Paris: Éditions du Seuil, 1979.

Efron, John M. *Defenders of the Race: Jewish Doctors and Race in Fin-de-siècle Europe*. New Haven CT: Yale University Press, 1994.

Ehrenreich, Barbara, and Deidre English. *For Her Own Good: Two Centuries of the Experts Advice to Women*. New York: Random House, 1978.

———. *Witches, Midwives, and Nurses: A History of Women Healers*. New York: Feminist Press, 2010.

El Ghoul, Yahya. *Naturalisation et Nationalisme en Tunisie de l'Entre-Deux-Guerres*. Tunis: Centre de Publication Universitaire, 2009.

Eloy, G. *La Ville de Tunis à l'Exposition Coloniale Internationale de 1931*. Tunis: Imprimerie Ch. Weber, 1931.

Faivre d'Arcier, Jeanne. *Habiba Messika: La brûlure du péché*. Paris: Belfond, 1998.

Falk, R. "Zionism and the Biology of the Jews." *Science in Context* 11, no. 3–4 (Autumn–Winter 1998): 587–607.

Fellous, Sonia, ed. *Juifs et musulmans de Tunisie: Fraternité et déchirements*. Paris: Somogy édition d'art, 2003.

Fijalkow, Yankel. *La construction des ilôts insalubres: Paris 1850–1945*. Paris: L'Harmattan 1998.

Fischer-Tiné, Harald, and Michael Mann, eds. *Colonialism as Civilizing Mission: Cultural Ideology in British India*. London: Anthem Press, 2004.

Fortescue, William. *The Third Republic in France, 1870–1940*. London: Routledge, 2000.

Gallagher, Nancy. *Medicine and Power in Tunisia, 1780–1900*. Cambridge: Cambridge University Press, 1983.

Ganiage, J. *La crise des finances tunisiennes et l'ascension des juifs de Tunis*. Algiers: Imprimerie Rapide, 1955.

———. *Les origins du Protectorat français en Tunisie (1861–1891)*. Paris: Presses universitaires de France, 1959.

Gaumer, Benoît. *L'organisation sanitaire en Tunisie sous le protectorat français (1881–1956)*. Laval, Québec: Presses de l'Université de Laval, 2006.

Gikandi, Simon. "Picasso, Africa, and the Schemata of Difference." *Modernism/Modernity* 10, no. 3 (2003): 455–80.

Gilman, Sander. *Difference and Pathology: Stereotypes of Sexuality, Race, and Madness*. Ithaca NY: Cornell University Press, 1985.

———. *The Jew's Body*. London: Routledge, 1991.

Goldstein, Jan E. *Console and Classify: The French Psychiatric Professor in the Nineteenth Century*. Cambridge: Cambridge University Press, 1987.

Gottriech, Emily. "Historicizing the Concept of Arab Jews in the Maghrib." *Jewish Quarterly Review* 98, no. 4 (2008): 433–51.

———. *The Mellah of Marrakesh: Jewish and Muslim Space in Morocco's Red City*. Bloomington: Indiana University Press, 2007.

———. "Rethinking the 'Islamic City' from the Perspective of Jewish Space." *Jewish Social Studies* 11, no. 1 (2004): 118–46.

Graetz, Michael. *The Jews in Nineteenth Century France: From the French Revolution to the Alliance Israelite Universelle*. Palo Alto CA: Stanford University Press, 1996.

Green, Arnold H. *The Tunisian Ulama 1873–1915, Social Structure and Response to Ideological Currents*. Leiden: E. J. Brill, 1978.

Green, Nancy. *The Pletzl of Paris: Jewish Immigrant Workers in the Belle Époque*. New York: Holmes & Meier, 1986.

Grégoire, Henri. *Essai sur la régénération physique, morale et politique des Juifs: ouvrage couronné par la Société Royale des Sciences et des Arts de Metz, le 23 août 1788*. Paris: Flammarion, 1988.

———. *Motion en faveur des Juifs*. Vol. 3 of *La Révolution Française et l'émancipation des Juifs*. 1788. Reprint, Paris: Editions d'Histoire Sociale, 1968.

Gross, L. "How Charles Nicolle of the Pasteur Institute Discovered That Epidemic Typhus Is Transmitted by Lice: Reminiscences from My Years at the Pasteur

Institute in Paris." *Proceedings of the National Academy of Sciences of the United States of America* 93, no. 20 (1996): 10539–40.

Hagège, Claude, and Bernard Zarca. "Les Juifs et la France en Tunisie: les bénéfices d'une relation triangulaire." *Le Mouvement Social* 4, no. 197 (October–December 2001): 9–28.

Hamrouni, Ahmed. *Habiba M'skia: Artiste accomplice*. Tunis: L'Univers du livre, 2007.

Hart, Michael B. *The Healthy Jew: The Symbiosis of Judaism and Modern Medicine*. Cambridge: Cambridge University Press, 2007.

Haskell, Thomas L., ed. *The Authority of Experts: Studies in History and Theory*. Bloomington: Indiana University Press, 1984.

Hazbun, Waleed. *Beaches, Ruins, Resorts: The Politics of Tourism in the Arab World*. Minneapolis: University of Minnesota Press, 2008.

Heap, Chad C. *Slumming: Sexual and Racial Encounters in American Nightlife, 1885–1940*. Chicago: Chicago University Press, 2009.

Herzl, Theodor. *Der Judenstaat*. Bremen: Faksimile-Verlag/Versand, 1984.

Hesse-Wartegg, Ernstt von. *Tunis, Land und Leute*. Vienna: A. Hartleben, 1882.

Hunt, Lynn. "French History in the Last Twenty Years: The Rise and Fall of the *Annales* Paradigm." *Journal of Contemporary History* 27, no. 2 (April 1986): 209–24.

Hunt, Nancy Rose. *A Colonial Lexicon: Of Birth Ritual, Medicalization, and Mobility in the Congo*. Durham NC: Duke University Press, 1999.

Huysmann, J.-K. *A rebours*. Paris: Bibiotheque Charpentier, 1921.

Hyman, Paula. *The Emancipation of the Jews of Alsace: Acculturation and Tradition in the Nineteenth Century*. New Haven CT: Yale University Press, 1991.

———. *From Dreyfus to Vichy: The Remaking of French Jewry, 1906–1939*. New York: Columbia University Press, 1979.

———. *Gender and Assimilation in Modern Jewish History: The Roles and Representations of Women*. Seattle: University of Washington Press, 1995.

———. *The Jews of Modern France*. Berkeley: University of California Press, 1998.

Jackson, Peter. "Post-War Politics and the Historiography of French Strategy and Diplomacy Before the Second World War." *History Compass* 4, no. 5 (2006): 870–905.

Jacob, Margaret C. *The Cultural Meaning of the Scientific Revolution*. Philadelphia: Temple University Press, 1988.

Jolly, Margaret. "Introduction." In *Maternities and Modernities: Colonial and Postcolonial Experiences in Asia and the Pacific*, edited by Kalpana Ram and Margaret Jolly. Cambridge: Cambridge University Press, 1998.

Jordan, David P. "Haussmann and Haussmannisation: The Legacy for Paris." *French Historical Studies* 27, no. 1 (Winter 2004): 87–113.

Jordan, Nicole. *The Popular Front and Central Europe: The Dilemmas of French Impotence, 1918–1940*. Cambridge: Cambridge University Press, 1992.

Kabbani, Rana. *Imperial Fictions: Europe's Myths of Orient*. London: Pandora Press, 1994.

Kalman, Samuel. "Fascism and Algérianité: The *Croix de Feu* and the Indigenous Question in 1930s Algeria." In *The French Colonial Mind*, vol. 2, edited by Martin Thomas, 124–28. Lincoln: University of Nebraska Press, 2011.

Kaplan, Marion A. *The Making of the Jewish Middle Class: Women, Family, and Identity in Imperial Germany*. New York: Oxford University Press, 1991.

Kassab, Ahmed. "La communauté israélite de Tunisie entre la francisation et le sionisme (1930–1940)." In *Les Mouvements politiques et sociaux dans la Tunisie des années 1930*, edited by Moncef Chenoufi, 525–48. Tunis: Ministere de l'Education, de l'Enseignement et de la Recherche Scientifique, 1987.

Katz, Ethan B. "Between Emancipation and Persecution." *Journal of North African Studies* 17, no. 5 (2012): 793–820.

Kazdaghli, Habib. "L'évolution organisationnelle du mouvement communiste en Tunisie (1926–1939)." In *Les Mouvements politiques et sociaux dans la Tunisie des années 1930*, edited by Moncef Chenoufi, 203–20. Tunis: Ministere de l'Education, de l'Enseignement et de la Recherche Scientifique, 1987.

Keller, Richard. *Colonial Madness: Psychiatry in French North Africa*. Chicago: University of Chicago, 2007.

Kenbib, Mohammed. *Juifs et Musulmans au Maroc, 1859–1948*. Rabat: Faculté des lettres et des sciences humaines, 1994.

Klaus, Alisa. *Every Child a Lion: The Origins of Maternal and Infant Health Policy in the United States and France, 1890–1920*. Ithaca NY: Cornell University Press, 1993.

Kruger, Steven F. *The Spectral Jew: Conversion and Embodiment in Medieval Europe*. Minneapolis: University of Minnesota Press, 2006.

Kuhn, Thomas. *The Structure of Scientific Revolutions*. Chicago: University of Chicago Press, 1962.

Kuperminc, Jean-Claude. "Le Regard des Premiers Instituteurs de l'Alliance." In *Entre Occident et Orient*, edited by Denis Cohen-Tannoudji, 347–56. Paris: Edition de l'Eclat, 2003.

Laloum, Jean. "Entre aryanisation et déportations." In *Vivre et survivre dans le Marais: au coeur de Paris du moyen âge à nos jours*, edited by Jean-Pierre Azéma, 367–90. Paris: Editions le Manuscrit, 2005.

Land, Joy. "Corresponding Lives: Women Educators of the Alliance Israélite Universelle School for Girls in the City of Tunis, 1882–1914." PhD diss., University of California, Los Angeles, 2006.

Laqueur, Thomas. *Making Sex: Body and Gender from the Greeks to Freud*. Cambridge MA: Harvard University Press, 1992.

Larguèche, Abdelhamid. *Les ombres de Tunis: marginaux et minorités aux XVIIIème et XIXème siècles*. Paris: Arcantères, 2000.

Laskier, Michael. *The Alliance Israélite Universelle and the Jewish Communities of Morocco, 1862–1962*. Albany: State University of New York Press, 1983.

———. "Aspects of the Activities of the Alliance Israelite Universelle in the Jewish Communities of the Middle East and North Africa: 1860–1918." *Modern Judaism* 3, no. 2 (May 1983): 147–71.

———. "The Evolution of Zionist Activity in the Jewish Communities of Morocco, Tunisia, and Algeria: 1897–1947." *Studies in Zionism* 4 (1987): 205–36.

———. *North African Jewry in the Twentieth Century: The Jews of Morocco, Tunisia, and Algeria*. New York: NYU Press, 1994.

Latour, Bruno. *The Pasteurization of France*. Translated by Alan Sheridan and John Law. Cambridge MA: Harvard University Press, 1986.

———. *We Have Never Been Modern*. Cambridge MA: Harvard University Press, 1991.

Lauzel, M. "Un étrange quartier de Paris." *Revue de Paris*, t. 1 (1912): 777–93.

Lehmann, Matthias B. "A Livornese 'Port Jew' and the Sephardim of the Ottoman Empire." *Jewish Social Studies* 11, no. 2 (Winter 2005): 51–76.

Le Pautremat, Pascal, and Charles-Robert Ageron. *La politique musulmane de la France au XXe siècle. De l'Hexagone aux terres d'Islam: espoirs, réussites, échecs*. Paris: Maisonneuve et Larose, 2003.

Levy, Lital. "Historicizing the Concept of Arab Jews in the Mashriq." *Jewish Quarterly Review* 98, no. 4 (2008): 452–69.

Lewis, Mary D. *Divided Rule: Sovereignty and Empire in French Tunisia, 1881–1938*. Berkeley: University of California Press, 2013.

Litt, Jacquelyn S. *Medicalized Motherhood: Perspectives from the Lives of African-American and Jewish Women*. Piscataway NJ: Rutgers University Press, 2000.

Lorcin, Patricia M. E. *Imperial Identities*. London: I. B. Tauris, 1995. Reprint, New York: St. Martin's Press, 1999.

———. *Kabyles, Arabs, Français: identités colonials*. Limoges: PULIM, 2005.

———. "Teaching Women and Gender in France d'Outre-Mer: Problems and Strategies." *French Historical Studies* 27, no. 2 (Spring 2004): 294–96.

Lowe, Lisa. *Critical Terrains: French and British Orientalisms*. Ithaca NY: Cornell University Press, 1992.

Lowney, Chris. *A Vanished World: Muslims, Christians, and Jews in Medieval Spain*. Oxford: Oxford University Press, 2006.

Lyons, Jonathan. *The House of Wisdom: How the Arabs Transformed Western Civilization*. London: Bloomsbury, 2010.

Magri, Susanna, and Christian Topalov. "L'habitat du salarié moderne en France, Grande-Bretagne, Italie, et aux Etats-Unis, 1910–1925." In *Les chantiers de la paix sociale (1900–1940)*, edited by Yves Cohen and Rémi Baudoui, 223–54. Fontenay/Saint-Cloud: ENS Editions, 1995.

Majhoubi, Ali. *Les Origines du mouvement national en Tunisie (1904–1934)*. Tunis: Université de Tunis, 1982.

Malinas, M., and M. Tostivint. "Mutualité coöperative et projet général d'assistance médicale indigène en Tunisie, III. Socialisation de la médicine et de la pharmacie par la mutualité coöpérative. Project général d'assistance médicale et pharmaceutique en Tunisie." *Revue tunisienne* (1905): 480–515.

Maltzan, Heinrich Freiherr von. *Reise in den Regenschaften Tunis und Tripolis*. Vol. 1. Leipzig: Veit, 1870.

Mandel, Maud. *Muslims and Jews in France: History of a Conflict*. Princeton NJ: Princeton University Press, 2014.

Manderson, Lenore. "Shaping Reproduction." In *Maternities and Modernities: Colonial and Postcolonial Experiences in Asia and the Pacific*, edited by Kalpana Ram and Margaret Jolly, 26–49. Cambridge: Cambridge University Press, 1998.

Marçais, Georges. *L'Architecture musulmane d'Occident: Tunisie, Algérie, Maroc, Espagne, Sicile*. Paris: Arts et Métiers Graphiques, 1954.

———. *L'art musulman*. Paris: Presses Universitaires de France, 1962.

Marcotte, Edmond. *L'art de batir une maison agreeable et saine: ouvrage fundamental sur la technique et l'hygiene des habitations et des Installations accessories dans les Villes et a la Campagne, en France et aux Colonies*. Paris: Librairie polytechnique Ch. Beranger, 1930.

Marcovich, Anne. "French Colonial Medicine and Colonial Rule: Algeria and Indochina." In *Disease, Medicine and Empire*, edited by Roy MacLeod and Milton Lewis, 103–17. New York: Routledge, 1988.

Marcus, Sharon. *Apartment Stories: City and Home in Nineteenth-Century Paris and London*. Berkeley: University of California Press, 1999.

Marrus, Michael R. *The Politics of Assimilation: A Study of the French Jewish Community at the Time of the Dreyfus Affair*. New York: Clarendon Press, 1971.

Maxwell, Richard. *The Mysteries of Paris and London*. Charlottesville: University Press of Virginia, 1992.

Menocal, Maria Rosa. *The Ornament of the World: How Muslims, Jews and Christians Created a Culture of Tolerance in Medieval Spain*. Boston: Back Bay Books, 2003.

Miller, Sarah Alison. *Medieval Monstrosity and the Female Body*. New York: Routledge, 2010.

Miller, Susan Gilson. "Apportioning Sacred Space in a Moroccan City: The Case of Tangier, 1860–1912." *City & Society* 13, no. 1 (2001): 57–83.

Miller, Susan Gilson, et al. "Inscribing Minority Space in the Islamic City: The Jewish Quarter of Fez (1438–1912)." *Journal of the Society of Architectural Historians* 60, no. 3 (September 2001): 310–27.

Miller, Susan Gilson, and Mauro Bertagnin. *The Architecture and Memory of the Minority Quarter in the Muslim Mediterranean City*. Cambridge MA: Harvard University Press, 2010.

Modena, M. Mayer. "The Spoken Languages of the Jews of Italy." In *The Jews of Italy: Memory and Identity*, edited by B. Garvin and B. Cooperman, 307–16. Bethesda: University Press of Maryland, 2000.

Monaco, C. S. "Port Jews or a People of the Diaspora? A Critique of the Port Jew Concept." *Jewish Social Studies* 15, no. 2 (Winter 2009): 137–66.

Morton, Patricia. *Hybrid Modernities: Architecture and Representation at the 1931 Colonial Exposition, Paris*. Cambridge MA: MIT University Press, 2003.

Motadel, David, ed. *Islam and the European Empires*. Oxford: Oxford University Press, 2014.

Muraud, Lion. *L'hygiene dans la Republique: la santé publique en France, ou, l'utopie contrariee (1870–1918)*. Paris: Fayard, 1996.

Nafafe, Jose Lingna. "Europe in Africa and Africa in Europe: Rethinking Postcolonial Space, Cultural Encounters, and Hybridity." *European Journal of Social Theory* 16, no. 1 (February 2012): 51–68.

Nahum, Henri. *Le médicine française et les Juifs, 1930–1945*. Paris: L'Harmattan, 2006.

Nash, Linda L. *Inescapable Ecologies: A History of Environment, Disease, and Knowledge*. Berkeley: University of California, 2006.

Necheles, Ruth. *The Abbé Grégoire, 1787–1831: The Odyssey of an Egalitarian*. Santa Barbara, CA: Praeger, 1971.

———. "The Abbé Grégoire's Work in Behalf of Jews, 1788–1791." *French Historical Studies* 6, no. 2 (Autumn 1969): 172–84.

Nordau, Max Simon. *Degeneration*. London: Heinemann, 1895.

Nye, Robert. *Crime, Madness, and Politics in Modern France: The Medical Concept of National Decline*. Princeton NJ: Princeton University Press, 1984.

———. "Degeneration, Neurasthenia and the Culture of Sport in Belle Époque France." *Journal of Contemporary History* 17, no. 1 (January 1982): 51–68.

Osborne, Michael A. *The Emergence of Tropical Medicine in France*. Chicago: University of Chicago Press, 2014.

Perkins, Kenneth. *A History of Modern Tunisia*. Cambridge: Cambridge University Press, 2004.

Perpetua, P. *Geografia della Reggenza di Tunisi*. Torino: G. B. Paravia, 1882.

Pick, Daniel. *Faces of Degeneration: A European Disorder, c.1848–1918*. Cambridge: Cambridge University Press, 1989.

Pilbeam, Pamela. "The Growth of Liberalism and the Crisis of the Bourbon Restoration, 1827–1830." *Historical Journal* 25 (1982): 351–66.

Prakash, Gyan. *Another Reason: Science and the Imagination of Modern India*. Princeton NJ: Princeton University Press, 1999.

Pratt, Mary Louise. "Arts of the Contact Zone." *Profession* (1991): 33–40.

———. *Imperial Eyes: Travel Writing and Transculturation*. London: Routledge, 1992.

Presner, Todd Samuel. *Muscular Judaism: The Jewish Body and the Politics of Regeneration*. London: Routledge, 2007.

Priestly, Herbert Ingram. *France Overseas: A Study of Modern Imperialism*. Berkeley: University of California Press, 1938.

Prochaska, David. *Making Algeria French: Colonialism in Bône, 1870–1920*. Cambridge: Cambridge University Press, 2004.

Proust, Marcel. *A la recherche du temps perdu*. Paris: Gallimard, 1913–27.

Rabinow, Paul. *French Modern: Norms and Forms of the Social Environment*. Cambridge MA: MIT Press, 1989.

Rauch, André. *Boxe, violence du XXe siècle*. Paris: Aubier, 1992.

Raymond, André. *Grandes villes arabes à l'époque ottoman*. Paris: Sindbad, 1985.

Revel, Jacques. *Jeux d'échelles: La micro-analyse à l'expérience*. Paris: Gallimard and Le Seuil, 1996.

Robert, Paul. "Nos édiles." *Nouvelle revue française* (1906): 57. Reprinted in Yankel Fijalkow, *La construction des ilôts insalubres: Paris 1850–1945*. Paris: L'Harmattan, 1998.

Rodrigue, Aron. *De l'Instruction à l'Emancipation*. Translated by Jacqueline Carnaud. Paris: Calman-Levy, 1989.

———. *French Jews, Turkish Jews: The Alliance Israélite Universelle and the Politics of Jewish Schooling in Turkey, 1860–1925*. Bloomington: Indiana University Press, 1990.

———. *Images of Sephardi and Eastern Jewries in Transition: The Teachers of the Alliance Israélite Universelle, 1860–1939*. Seattle: University of Washington Press, 1993.

Rollman, Wilfrid J. "Some Reflections on Recent Trends in the Study of Modern North African History." In *The Maghrib in Question: Essays in History and Historiography*, edited by Michel Le Gall and Kenneth Perkins, 62–80. Austin: University of Texas, 1997.

Ross, Kristen. *Fast Cars, Clean Bodies: Decolonization and the Reordering of French Culture*. Cambridge MA: MIT Press, 1995.

Royer, J., ed. *L'Urbanisme aux colonies et dans les pays tropicaux*. Vol. 1. La Charité-sur-Loire: Delaynce, 1932.

Saadoun, Haim. "L'influence du sionisme." In *Juifs et Musulmans en Tunisie: Fraternité et déchirements*, edited by Sonia Fellous, 219–29. Paris: Somogy, 2003.

———. "Tunisia." In *The Jews of the Middle East and North Africa in Modern Times*, edited by Reeva S. Simon et al., 454–57. New York: Columbia University Press, 2003.

———. "Zionism in Tunisia, 1918–1948." PhD diss., Hebrew University, 1992.

Said, Edward. *Culture and Imperialism*. New York: Vintage Books, 1993.

———. *Orientalism*. New York: Vintage Books, 1979.

Sait, Siraj, and Hilary Lim. *Land, Law and Islam: Property and Human Rights in the Muslim World*. London: Zed Books, 2006.

Sand, Shlomo. *The Invention of the Jewish People*. Translated by Yael Lotan. London: Verso, 2009.

Sarfati, Shimshon. *Tounis "El Khadra," Tunis "La Verte:" Traditions ancestrales, légendes et coutumes juives en Tunisie, 1881–1948*. Tel Aviv: Institut Haberman d'études littéraires, 1995.

Schechter, Ronald. *Obstinate Hebrews: Representations of Jews in France, 1715–1815*. Berkeley: University of California Press, 2003.

Schlör, Joachim. *Nights in the Big City: Paris, Berlin, London 1840–1930*. London: Reaktion, 1998.

Schneider, William H. *Quality and Quantity: The Quest for Biological Regeneration in Twentieth-Century France*. Cambridge: Cambridge University Press, 1990.

———. "Toward the Improvement of the Human Race: The History of Eugenics in France." *Journal of Modern History* 54 (June 1982): 268–91.

Schreier, Joshua. *Arabs of the Jewish Faith: The Civilizing Mission in Colonial Algeria*. New Brunswick NJ: Rutgers University Press, 2010.

———. *From Jewish Regeneration to Colonialism: The Ideology and Practice of Civilizing in France and Algeria, 1815–1870*. PhD diss., New York University, 2003.

———. "Napoleon's Long Shadow: Morality, Civilization, and Jews in France and Algeria." *French Historical Studies* 30 (1): 77–103.

Schroeter, Daniel. "The Jewish Quarter of the Moroccan City." In *New Horizons in Sephardic Studies*, edited by George K. Zucker and Yedida K. Stillman, 67–81. Albany: State University of New York Press, 1993.

———. "Jewish Quarters in the Arab-Islamic Cities of the Ottoman Empire." In *The Jews of the Ottoman Empire*, edited by Avigdor Levy, 287–300. Princeton NJ: Darwin Press, 1994.

———. *Merchants of Essaouira: Urban Society and Imperialism in Southwestern Morocco, 1844–1886*. Cambridge: Cambridge University Press, 1988.

———. "The Shifting Boundaries of Moroccan Jewish Identities," *Jewish Social Studies* 15, no. 1 (Fall 2008): 145–64.

———. *The Sultan's Jew: Morocco and the Sephardi World*. Palo Alto CA: Stanford University Press, 2002.

Schroeter, Daniel J., and Joseph Chetrit. "Emancipation and Its Discontents: Jewish at the Formative Period of Colonial Rule in Morocco." *Jewish Social Studies* 13, no. 1 (Fall 2006): 170–206.

Sebag, Paul. *La Hara de Tunis: L'évolution d'un ghetto*. Paris: Presses Universitaires de France, 1959.

———. *Histoire des Juifs de Tunisie: des origines à nos jours*. Paris: L'Harmattan, 1991.

———. *Tunis: histoire d'une ville*. Paris: L'Harmattan, 1998.

Sepinwall, Alyssa G. *The Abbé Grégoire and the French Revolution: The Making of Modern Universalism*. Berkeley: University of California Press, 2005.

Sessions, Jennifer. *By Sword and Plow: France and the Conquest of Algeria*. Cornell: Cornell University Press, 2011.

Shah, Nyan. *Contagious Divides: Epidemics and Race in San Francisco's Chinatown*. Berkeley: University of California Press, 2001.

Shanahan, Timothy. *The Evolution of Darwinism: Selection, Adaptation and Progress in Evolutionary Biology*. Cambridge: Cambridge University Press, 2004.

Shepard, Todd. *The Invention of Decolonization: The Algerian War and the Remaking of France*. Ithaca NY: Cornell University Press, 2008.

Sherman, Daniel J. "The Arts and Sciences of Colonialism." *French Historical Studies* 23, no. 4 (2000): 707–29.

Shulewitz, Malka. *The Forgotten Millions: The Modern Jewish Exodus from Arab Lands*. London: Bloomsbury, 1999.

Silberman, Paul. "An Investigation of the Schools Operated by the Alliance Israélite Universelle from 1862 to 1940." PhD diss., New York University, 1974.

Silver, Brian L. *The Ascent of Science*. New York: Oxford University Press, 1998.

Simonsen, Jane E. *Making Home Work: Domesticity and Native American Assimilation in the American West, 1860–1919*. Chapel Hill: University of North Carolina Press, 2006.

Slymovics, Susan. "Geographies of Jewish Tlemcen." *Journal of North African Studies* 5, no. 4 (Winter 2000): 81–96.

Snouissi, M. L. "Aux origines du mouvement sioniste en Tunisie à la veille de la Grande Guerre: création de l'Aghoudat-Sion et sa première scission." *Cahiers de Tunisie*, 44, no. 157/8 (1991): 225–74.

Sorkin, David. "The Port Jews: Notes toward a Social Type." *Journal of Jewish Studies* 50, no. 1 (Spring 1999): 87–97.

Soulmagnon, Georges. *La loi tunisienne du 1er juillet 1885 sur la propriété immobilière et le régime des livres fonciers*. Paris: Siry, 1933.

Sowerwine, Charles. *France since 1870: Culture, Politics and Society*. Basingstoke, England: Palgrave, 2001.

Spivak, Gayatri Chakrovorty. *A Critique of Postcolonial Reason: Toward a History of the Vanishing Point*. Cambridge MA: Harvard University Press, 1999.

Starr, Paul. *The Social Transformation of American Medicine: The Rise of a Sovereign Profession and the Making of a Vast Industry*. New York: Basic Books, 1982.

Steedman, Carolyn Kay. *Dust: The Archive and Cultural History*. New Brunswick NJ: Rutgers University Press, 2002.

Stillman, Norm. *The Jews of Arab Lands in Modern Times*. Lincoln: University of Nebraska Press, 1999.

Stoler, Laura Ann. *Along the Archival Grain: Epistemic Anxieties and Colonial Common Sense*. Princeton NJ: Princeton University Press, 2010.

———. *Carnal Knowledge and Imperial Power: Race and the Intimate in Colonial Rule*. Berkeley: University of California Press, 2002.

———. *Imperial Debris: On Ruins and Ruination*. Durham NC: Duke University Press, 2013.

———. *Race and the Education of Desire: Foucault's History of Sexuality and the Colonial Order of Things*. Durham NC: Duke University Press, 1995.

Taïeb, Jacques. "Évolution et comportement démographiques des Juifs de Tunisie sous le protectorat français (1881–1956)." *Population* 37, no. 4/5 (1982): 957.

———. "Grana (Livornese)." In *Encyclopedia of Jews in the Islamic World*, edited by Norman A. Stillman. Leiden: Brill, 2011.

Taylor, Greg. *The Law of the Land: The Advent of the Torrens System in Canada*. Toronto: University of Toronto Press, 2008.

Thomas, Martin. *The French Colonial Mind*. Vol. 2. Lincoln: University of Nebraska Press, 2011.

Tilley, Helen. *Africa as a Living Laboratory: Empire, Development, and the Problem of Scientific Knowledge, 1870–1950*. Chicago: University of Chicago Press, 2011.

Tobi, Yosef. "Flāḥ, Shalom." *Encyclopedia of Jews in the Islamic World*, edited by Norman A. Stillman. Leiden: Brill, 2011.

Tomes, Nancy. *The Gospel of Germs: Men, Women, and the Microbe in American Life*. Cambridge MA: Harvard University Press, 1998.

Topalov, Christian. *Le logement en France: histoire d'une marchandise impossible*. Paris: Press de la fondation des sciences politiques, 1987.

Udovitch, Abraham, and Lucette Valensi. *The Last Arab Jews: The Communities of Jerba, Tunisia*. New York: Harwood Academic, 1984.

Ulrich, Laurel Thatcher. *The Life of Martha Ballard, Based on Her Diary, 1785–1812.* New York: Vintage Books, 1991.
Valensi, Lucette, and Nathan Wachtel. *Jewish Memories.* Translated by Barbara Harshav. Berkeley: University of California Press, 1991.
Vassel, Eusèbe. *Le Juif Tunisien.* Paris: Revue Indigène, 1907.
Vogel, Morris J., and Charles E. Rosenberg, eds. *The Therapeutic Revolution.* Philadelphia: University of Pennsylvania Press, 1979.
Voligny, R. Bouquero de. *À Tunis: Derrière les Murs.* Tunis: Guenard & Franchi, 1922.
White, Owen, and J. P. Daughton, eds. *In God's Empire: French Missionaries and the Modern World.* Oxford: Oxford University Press, 2012.
Wilder, Gary. *The French Imperial Nation-State: Negritude and Colonial Humanism between the Two Wars.* Chicago: University of Chicago Press, 2005.
Winock, Michel. *Histoire de l'extrême droite en France.* Paris: Seuil, 1994.
———. *Nationalisme, fascism et antisémitisme en France.* Paris: Seuil, 1990.
Winter, James. *London's Teeming Streets, 1830–1914.* London: Routledge, 1993.
Worboys, Michael. *Spreading Germs: Disease Theories and Medical Practice in Britain, 1865–1900.* Cambridge: University of Cambridge Press, 2000.
Wright, Gwendolyn. *The Politics of Design in French Colonial Urbanism.* Chicago: University of Chicago Press, 1991.
———. "Tradition in the Service of Modernity: Architecture and Urbanism in French Colonial Policy, 1900–1930." In *Tensions of Empire: Colonial Cultures in a Bourgeois World,* edited by Frederick Cooper and Ann Laura Stoler, 322–45. Berkeley: University of California Press, 1997.
Young, P. "Why Did the Torrens System Succeed in Australia yet Fail in North America?" *Australian Property Law Journal* 2 (1994): 228.
Zack, Lizabeth. "French and Algerian Identity Formation in 1890s Algeria." *French Colonial History* 2 (2002): 115–43.
Zarca, Bernard. *Une enfance juive tunisoise.* Paris: L'Harmattan, 2005.
Zola, Emile. *L'Assomoir.* Paris: Bibiothèque Charpentier, 1877.
———. *La bête humaine.* Paris: Bibiothèque Charpentier, 1890.
———. *Nana.* Paris: Bibiothèque Charpentier, 1880.
———. *Pot-bouille.* Paris: Imprimerie Emile Martinet, 1882.

INDEX

Page numbers in italic indicate illustrations.

IN THE FRANCE OVERSEAS SERIES

Regeneration through Empire: French Pronatalists and Colonial Settlement in the Third Republic
Margaret Cook Andersen

To Hell and Back: The Life of Samira Bellil
Samira Bellil
Translated by Lucy R. McNair
Introduction by Alec G. Hargreaves

Colonial Metropolis: The Urban Grounds of Anti-Imperialism and Feminism in Interwar Paris
Jennifer Anne Boittin

Paradise Destroyed: Catastrophe and Citizenship in the French Caribbean
Christopher M. Church

The French Navy and the Seven Years' War
Jonathan R. Dull

I, Nadia, Wife of a Terrorist
Baya Gacemi

Transnational Spaces and Identities in the Francophone World
Edited by Hafid Gafaïti, Patricia M. E. Lorcin, and David G. Troyansky

Contesting French West Africa: Battles over Schools and the Colonial Order, 1900–1950
Harry Gamble

The French Army and Its African Soldiers: The Years of Decolonization
Ruth Ginio

French Colonialism Unmasked: The Vichy Years in French West Africa
Ruth Ginio

Bourdieu in Algeria: Colonial Politics, Ethnographic Practices, Theoretical Developments
Edited and with an introduction by Jane E. Goodman and Paul A. Silverstein

Endgame 1758: The Promise, the Glory, and the Despair of Louisbourg's Last Decade
A. J. B. Johnston

French Mediterraneans: Transnational and Imperial Histories
Edited and with an introduction by Patricia M. E. Lorcin and Todd Shepard

The Cult of the Modern: Trans-Mediterranean France and the Construction of French Modernity
Gavin Murray-Miller

Cinema in an Age of Terror: North Africa, Victimization, and Colonial History
Michael F. O'Riley

Medical Imperialism in French North Africa: Regenerating the Jewish Community of Colonial Tunis
Richard C. Parks

Making the Voyageur World: Travelers and Traders in the North American Fur Trade
Carolyn Podruchny

A Workman Is Worthy of His Meat: Food and Colonialism in Gabon
Jeremy Rich

The Moroccan Soul: French Education, Colonial Ethnology, and Muslim Resistance, 1912–1956
Spencer D. Segalla

Silence Is Death: The Life and Work of Tahar Djaout
Julija Šukys

The French Colonial Mind, Volume 1: Mental Maps of Empire and Colonial Encounters
Edited and with an introduction by Martin Thomas

The French Colonial Mind, Volume 2: Violence, Military Encounters, and Colonialism
Edited and with an introduction by Martin Thomas

Beyond Papillon: The French Overseas Penal Colonies, 1854–1952
Stephen A. Toth

Madah-Sartre: The Kidnapping, Trial, and Conver(sat/s)ion of Jean-Paul Sartre and Simone de Beauvoir
Written and translated by Alek Baylee Toumi
With an introduction by James D. Le Sueur

CPSIA information can be obtained
at www.ICGtesting.com
Printed in the USA
LVOW07*0617060817
544007LV00002B/10/P

9 780803 268456